HERE'S WHAT THE EXPERTS SAY ABOUT
Get off the Menopause Roller Coaster:

"*Get off the Menopause Roller Coaster* offers many solutions that can greatly ease the symptoms of menopause. This is a fascinating book that every woman (and those who care about her) should read when she reaches this time in her life."
—MELVYN R. WERBACH, M.D., author of *Textbook of Nutritional Medicine*

"*Get off the Menopause Roller Coaster* is an absolute must for anyone seeking natural solutions to make the transition into menopause easier. Dr. Lieberman has done a superb job of helping women understand and treat the symptoms of menopause. This is the most thorough book of its kind."
—ALLAN MAGAZINER, D.O., Medical Director, Magaziner Center for Wellness and Anti-Aging, Cherry Hill, New Jersey, and author of *Total Health Handbook: Your Complete Wellness Resource* and *The Complete Idiot's Guide to Living Longer and Healthier*

"A concise, practical guide to natural alternatives for treating the symptoms of menopause from America's premier complementary nutritionist."
—RON HOFFMAN, M.D., Medical Director, The Hoffman Center, New York City, and author of *Intelligent Medicine*

Get Off
the
Menopause
Roller Coaster

Natural Solutions for
Mood Swings, Hot Flashes,
Fatigue, Anxiety, Depression,
and Other Symptoms

Shari Lieberman, Ph.D.

Avery
A MEMBER OF PENGUIN PUTNAM INC.
NEW YORK

Every effort has been made to ensure that the information contained in this book is complete and accurate. However, neither the publisher nor the author is engaged in rendering professional advice or services to the individual reader. The ideas, procedures, and suggestions contained in this book are not intended as a substitute for consulting with your physician. All matters regarding health require medical supervision. Neither the author nor the publisher shall be liable or responsible for any loss, injury, or damage allegedly arising from any information or suggestion in this book.

Most Avery books are available at special quantity discounts for bulk purchase for sales promotions, premiums, fund-raising, and educational needs. Special books or book excerpts also can be created to fit specific needs. For details, write Putnam Special Markets, 375 Hudson Street, New York, NY 10014.

Avery
a member of
Penguin Putnam Inc.
375 Hudson Street
New York, NY 10014
www.penguinputnam.com

Library of Congress Cataloging-in-Publication Data

Lieberman, Shari.
Get off the menopause roller coaster: natural solutions for mood swings, hot flashes, fatigue, anxiety, depression, and other symptoms/by Shari Lieberman.
p. cm.
Includes index.
ISBN 1-58333-000-3
1. Menopause—Complications—Alternative treatment. 2. Premenstrual syndrome—Alternative treatment. I. Title.
RG186.L46 2000
618.1'7506—dc21   00-023742

Printed in the United States of America

1 3 5 7 9 10 8 6 4 2

Cover design by Jack Ribik
Book design by Patrice Sheridan

Acknowledgments

A very special thanks to Batya Swift Yasgur. She has been the moving force who saw this project through from beginning to end. Without her, this book would not have been written.

Kudos and special thanks to Rudy Shur: friend, publisher, visionary. He has stood behind me and my work in every conceivable way.

Many thanks to Joanne Abrams for her keen eye for detail and her great organizational skills.

To my husband, Augusto,
whose love, support, and patience
make enormous projects possible

Contents

Introduction

You're a woman. I'm a woman. And as women, we're going to go through menopause. At some point in our lives, we will stop having menstrual periods. How will we approach this major milestone in our lives? If we are like most Western women, we may be looking toward menopause with dread. We may anticipate an array of unpleasant symptoms that are said to accompany the "change of life." But is that really necessary? Is this natural part of our life cycle really something we should be regarding with fear, as if we were headed toward a disease? Or can we adopt a different attitude, one that sees menopause as a time of health and vibrancy?

I firmly believe that menopause isn't something to fear. It isn't a disease. It's a time of life in which our bodies can grow healthier, stronger, and more vibrant. This book will show you how you can turn menopause into a health-enhancing experience.

Who I Am, and Why I Wrote This Book

As a woman, I'm tired of seeing menopause treated as a disease in the United States. I've traveled through Asia and discovered that Asian women do not experience those symptoms we commonly associate with menopause—hot flashes, vaginal dryness, and so on. My associations with these women, my study of the scientific research, and my clinical experience as a practicing nutritionist have convinced me that menopause is simply a transition that can be accompanied by good health and personal growth.

In my practice, I have seen too many American women who are afflicted by menopause and its accompanying set of symptoms. They are ravaged by mood swings, fatigue, headaches, hot flashes, and vaginal discomfort. Many of them have had hormones prescribed to them by their gynecologists and are taking hormone replacement therapy. When they come to me, they are surprised and disturbed that their symptoms have continued—even worsened—despite the hormones. Even more disturbing, many have developed additional symptoms and problems, such as breast or uterine cancer. The contrast between my American patients and the Asian women I've encountered in my travels is staggering.

Here's the good news: With some simple, inexpensive, and noninvasive dietary supplements, you can avoid the unpleasant symptoms and emerge from this stage of life in even better health than you were before!

How Can This Book Help You?

If you are reading these words, you are probably a woman over age forty who is beginning to look toward the physical changes that lie ahead for you in the coming years. Maybe you are already experiencing some changes: fatigue, which you can't attribute just to lack of sleep; unusual irritability, and not only at "that time of the month"; an irregular menstrual cycle, or staining between periods.

Or maybe you are farther along in the process, already experiencing hot flashes or vaginal dryness. Your gynecologist is recommending hormone replacement therapy. You're confused. You're scared. You've heard that some of the symptoms can be controlled with estrogen. You've been told that estrogen will also keep you younger and prevent such conditions as osteoporosis. It's tempting, but does it work? And is it safe?

This book will answer your questions about hormone replacement therapy. And what's more important, it will guide you through a natural, safe, and effective menopause program that will address all your concerns. This program includes physical as well as emotional aspects. You will learn what to eat and also what to avoid—particularly about the use of phytohormones (plant hormones) as alternatives to conventional hormone replacement therapy. You will learn about herbs, vitamins, and other supplements that can address your symptoms: where to obtain them, what quantities and types to take, and what dosages. You will learn how to incorporate your supplements into a healthy program that includes exercise and emotional support.

Issues Covered in This Book

Chapter 1 defines menopause and explains what is happening in your body during this time in your life. It lists some of the most common symptoms, and explains why they occur. It also touches upon more serious problems, such as osteoporosis, heart disease, and changes in sexual function.

Chapter 2 focuses on conventional hormone replacement therapy, particularly the estrogen-replacement myth and the progestin controversy. It evaluates the claim that hormone replacement therapy (HRT) can enhance health, reduce symptoms, and keep women younger for longer. It describes the often-underplayed dangers involved in the use of synthetic hormones, and introduces readers to the concept of natural hormones.

Chapter 3 introduces phytohormones as part of a comprehensive dietary menopause program. It lists the various names and sources of these plant hormones, and how they can be incorporated into your diet.

In chapter 4 you will be introduced to the various nutritional supplements that address menopausal symptoms. The chapter lists and describes these items. It provides guidance regarding where you can obtain them, in which form they should be taken, which symptoms they address, and which dosages are most effective. The handy, easy-reference tables at the back of the chapter will help you choose supplements that address your particular constellation of discomforts and concerns.

Chapter 5 teaches you about exercise. You will learn how to exercise and—equally important—how *not* to exercise. You will learn which exercises contribute to healthy bones, which strengthen the heart, and which can most easily be integrated into your lifestyle.

Growing older often raises issues for women—especially American women—regarding their desirability, sexuality, and usefulness as members of society. Chapter 6 looks at your attitudes and feelings, exploring self-defeating beliefs about aging, and suggesting avenues to explore so as to feel optimistic, cheerful, and happy about the new phase of life you are entering.

If you continue to wonder whether hormone replacement therapy will help you, or find that none of the suggestions in chapters 3, 4, 5, and 6 have been sufficient to remedy your symptoms, you can revisit the subject of hormones in chapter 7. You will learn how to find out with scientific precision exactly which hormones you lack, and how to correct your imbalances.

Finally, chapter 8 will provide you with some suggestions to help you implement this transformative health program—whatever your particular stage in the menopausal process, and whatever your symptoms might be.

At the back of the book you will find references, suggestions for further reading, and resources to help you locate products or services discussed in the book.

How to Use This Book

If you are currently experiencing uncomfortable symptoms, you should begin with the chart at the end of chapter 4. You don't need to read everything in order to start experiencing immediate relief! The supplements on the chart are safe and effective if you follow the recommended dosages. If you want to understand more about the recommended product—let's say you've never heard of black cohosh and you want to find out what it is—you can turn to the entry earlier in chapter 4.

If your doctor has recommended hormone replacement therapy, you can educate yourself about your options by reading chapters 2 and 7, and then make a reasoned and informed decision.

If you're a woman looking toward menopause within the coming years but are not yet experiencing any particular symptoms or problems, I would advise you to read this book cover to cover. You will then understand what menopause is and how you can build your health even prior to menopause. No matter what your stage in life, if you begin to adopt the lifestyle changes I suggest in this book, your health will improve and you will thrive.

Feeling Younger While Growing Older

In the United States, we tend to regard aging with horror. We believe that to grow older means to lose our good health, energy, passion, vitality, and sexuality. I'm here to tell you that nothing could be further from the truth. You can retain your vigor, love of life, and attractiveness. You can grow older and feel even younger than you did when you were young! This book will help you to do so. I wish you success, vibrancy, and joy.

One

Understanding Menopause:
Is Menopause a Disease?

What do you think of when you hear the word *menopause?* Do you think of a network of common symptoms and conditions, such as hot flashes, fatigue, or vaginal dryness? If you are like most Western women, you think of a period of time often called "the change," during which the body is undergoing a series of unpleasant transitions. In truth, however, the word *menopause* simply means the "pause of the menses"—the last menstrual period. The stages preceding that final milestone and following it are certainly fraught with changes, both physical and emotional, but those changes are poorly understood and often unnecessary.

It's sad for me to hear the misconceptions and folklore—as ungrounded as old wives' tales—that most women accept as gospel. This chapter will address some common misunderstandings associated with menopause. It will explain what menopause is, and also what it isn't, defining some essential terms that are often misused. You will learn about the physiological changes that occur before and during menopause, the psychological and emotional adjustments that are called for, the stages of menopause, and the bodily experiences associated with each of those stages. Please note that I am using the words *bodily experiences* rather than *symptoms*, because all too often we associate *symptoms* with disease, and my contention is that menopause is not a disease. It is a natural and healthy process, something we can look forward to, instead of dreading. In other cultures, the time preceding and following menopause is regarded with reverence and respect. Unfortunately, all too many of us associate it with illness, discomfort, and degeneration—an attitude I hope to change with this book.

This chapter will touch upon some of the problems that concern women undergoing the menopausal transition as well as women who have already completed menopause. These problems include heart disease, osteoporosis, and sexual dysfunction. We will also look at general attitudes toward menopause and how these might affect your own experience of this important milestone.

What Happens in the Body During Menopause?

You were born with some two million eggs in your ovaries. The ovaries are organs located on either side of your pelvic region, in your lower abdomen. These eggs, nestled in egg follicles, lay dormant and immature until you reached puberty, when your body started changing and producing hormones. At that time, about four hundred to five hundred had matured and were ready to be released.

Once you reached *menarche*—the advent of your first menstrual period—you entered your reproductive years, and your body began its monthly cycles (after an adjustment period of a few months of irregular menstrual appearances). During the early part of the menstrual cycle, your body prepared for possible pregnancy. The pituitary gland, located in your head, released hormones called FSH (follicle stimulating hormone) and LH (leutenizing hormone). These caused the egg follicles in your ovaries to ripen, and one of them to become a full-grown egg. The follicle began to produce two essential female hormones: estrogen and progesterone, with estrogen dominating during the early part of the cycle and progesterone taking over during the second part of the cycle. The estrogen caused your uterine lining to thicken to provide a cushion for a fertilized egg that might attach itself and grow into an embryo, then a fetus, then a baby. It caused the egg follicle to rupture, releasing the egg.

So once a month, an egg began its journey from your ovary to your uterus. It traveled along the fallopian tube to the uterus, where it impatiently waited for a sperm to fertilize it. This second part of the menstrual cycle, called *ovulation,* was characterized by an increase in the production of a hormone called *progesterone.* If your egg was not fertilized, progesterone caused the uterus to shed its lining, which was then released through the vagina. That is the process known as menstruation.

As you approach the end of your reproductive years and the beginning of menopause, the number of eggs in your ovaries starts to diminish. This process, which begins during your mid-thirties, begins to accelerate by your late forties. There are several reasons: one is the natural aging process. Eggs have their own life span that sooner or later runs out. Hereditary factors, illness, stress, and environmental toxins can contribute to a more rapid destruction of the eggs. The result is a sharp decrease in estrogen and progesterone production, leading to a host of physical occurrences, and culminating in the complete cessation of menstruation.

This, friends, is something to be grateful for, rather than to resist. Do you really want to be pregnant in your fifties or sixties? The dropping of estrogen levels and the resultant cessation of menstruation are a blessing! For many women, the time following menopause brings sexual awakening because they no longer have to worry about birth control, pregnancy, or spontaneity. The kids are usually old enough to be somewhat independent, and so romance and lovemaking can be prioritized in ways that were not possible earlier. In chapter 6, we will discuss attitude and how you can regard menopause as a plus, rather than a minus.

Now that we know what menopause is, let's take a more careful look at how it proceeds—what happens first, what happens next, and what you might expect.

What Are the Stages of Menopause?

Menopause is a milestone preceded by stages. It does not happen all at once. As the eggs gradually die off and estrogen levels begin to drop, the changes begin to occur. They can creep up gradually, during a lengthy period of time—perhaps as long as ten years. This phase is called *perimenopause,* or the *climacteric.* For some women, the process begins in the thirties; other women begin this phase in their forties. At first, you might experience fatigue, irregular periods, spotting or staining between periods, or an unusually heavy flow. Your cycle will change as well. Your periods may be closer together, or farther apart. They may be lighter, heavier, or just different. You may experience some mild sleep disturbances or just the occasional sensation of feeling "off" and not quite yourself. Your body is setting the stage for the more dramatic changes that lie ahead. We'll look at these changes below.

Menopause—the cessation of the menses—follows perimenopause. There is a final menstrual period. It is usually different from other periods— it may be shorter or longer, heavier or lighter. Time to give away those annoying pads and tampons! And time to look at the years ahead, the postmenopausal years, and some of the health challenges, such as heart disease and osteoporosis, that all too often accompany the aging process of American women.

Common Perimenopausal Conditions and Experiences

During the years preceding that final menstrual period, the reproductive system closes up shop. The hormonal changes responsible for the tapering off and ending of reproductive possibility often lead to uncomfortable physical experiences, as the body adjusts to new hormonal levels. You might notice some or all of several occurrences. Not all women experience all the events described below, but most of them are fairly common to the majority of Western women. In fact, according to Dr. Carolyn De-Marco, author of *Take Charge of Your Body*, 90 percent of American women experience some form of perimenopausal discomfort. As you go through the list of symptoms below, please bear in mind that the remainder of this book will address whether all these are actually intrinsic to perimenopause, or whether some can actually be avoided or curtailed.

Hot Flashes

The sudden sensation of intense heat and flushing affecting the upper part or all of the body is called a hot flash. It is probably the most common menopausal affliction, affecting some 60 percent of American menopausal women. In fact, the very word *menopause* often brings an immediate association with hot flashes. During a hot flash, there is a rush of heat to the face and neck, often accompanied by red blotches on the arms, chest, and back. As the heat wanes, the body must readjust its temperature—a process that can lead to sweating or chills. Hot flashes range in duration, lasting from a few moments to as long as half an hour, and occasionally even longer. As one patient's husband put it, "My wife takes her own little vacation to Bermuda several times each day!"

Hot flashes are not confined to daytime hours. They can strike at night as well. When they do, they take the form of night sweats that can awaken you just when you've finally drifted off to sleep. You wake up drenched, but feeling as though you are on fire. Some American women find themselves changing linens once or twice a night!

Mood Swings

Some women report severe mood swings, almost reminiscent of their adolescent years. They can be weepy and depressed one moment, anxious and jittery the next, cheerful and ebullient after that. The general feeling is that some alien force has taken over, leading to a sense of "strangeness," almost as if the selves they knew had ceased to exist. Some women are not quite sure what their mood will be from one day to the next, or exactly what will trigger the mood swings. In fact, for some of my patients, mood swings represent the most difficult and frustrating aspect of perimenopause. I hear the constant refrain "Dr. Lieberman, I feel so out of control!"

Fatigue

The tiredness and "draggy" feeling of the early stages of perimenopause can develop into a major sense of exhaustion as the process continues. Some of this tiredness can be attributed to the sleep changes that accompany hormonal fluctuations. Many women find their sleep disrupted by night sweats and are understandably groggy and bleary-eyed the next day. It's hard to feel alert, upbeat, and energetic when you're not sleeping well at night! It's even harder if you're addressing your sleeplessness through drugs that can lead to drowsiness, addiction, and mood changes.

Menstrual Changes

The menstrual cycle becomes increasingly irregular, with periods showing up back-to-back, or being delayed by several months. This is due to the hormonal fluctuations taking place in your body. The incidence of staining between periods usually increases. Some periods may be characterized by an unusually heavy flow or an unusual amount of discomfort. Many women who were "spoiled" by predictable and regular periods complain that they no longer know their own bodies or how to prepare themselves at the beginning of a workday or before an overnight trip. When will their period arrive? How long will it last? Will they have to take off from work, even though menstruation has never "gotten them down" before? "It's weird," said one of my patients. "I thought I knew myself. Now, I don't even know how to pack for vacation! I don't know whether to come equipped for my period or not. I don't know whether to bring a bathing suit because I may not feel well enough for swimming if I do get it. I've become a stranger to myself."

Vaginal Changes

As you progress through perimenopause, your vaginal walls might become progressively thinner and dryer. They also can lose their elasticity. These changes might make you more vulnerable to infections such as candida, which is a yeast infection. Vaginal dryness and thinning out can also affect your sexual experience, since intercourse might become uncomfortable or painful due to the lack of lubrication and the fragility of the vaginal wall.

Sexual Changes

The vaginal dryness mentioned above obviously has an impact on the sex drive. Who wants to engage in an activity that brings pain instead of pleasure? But there is another reason that some women experience diminished libido: Hormonal fluctuations can in and of themselves reduce the desire for sex. This is not only a physical but also a psychological phenomenon. American women have been taught that youth is synonymous with beauty and sexual attractiveness. As we age, we are often vulnerable to the media-promoted message that we are losing our sexuality, and we may respond by beginning to regard ourselves as asexual beings. One of the most common fears and complaints of the perimenopausal woman is that she no longer feels sensual.

Miscellaneous Symptoms

The symptoms below are less common than the ones described above but can be disconcerting and even debilitating at times. All of them can be attributed to the impact of changing hormonal levels.

Headaches   Many women experience headaches during the perimenopausal years. Most often, these are women who had already been subject to headaches, but during the years preceding menopause, their headaches strike with greater frequency and intensity.

Palpitations   Some women begin to experience palpitations, or a "fluttery feeling in the heart." These are not necessarily in and of themselves problematic unless you have a preexisting heart condition, but it is advisable to have a competent cardiologist assess the situation.

Joint Pain   If you are experiencing some achiness of the joints, you do not need to automatically assume that you are developing arthritis. Joints are among the most sensitive parts of the human body. Have you noticed that you ache all over when you have the flu? Have any of you experienced that flulike, achy feeling during your menstrual periods? Your joints are quick to respond to changes in body temperature, as well as changes in hormonal levels. They are barometers of change, letting you know that something is going on inside your body.

Burning Mouth   A small number of women experience a dry and burning mouth—an oral hot flash. If you find yourself wondering if you have a steam iron wedged between your tongue and your palate, don't worry. You can use the same simple and effective natural remedies for burning mouth as you use for hot flashes.

Digestive Changes   Some women experience bloating, flatulence, and indigestion—all caused by the hormonal roller-coaster effect and its impact on digestive enzymes. Have you ever felt nauseated or queasy right before or during your period? Remember the morning sickness you experienced during the early months of your pregnancy? Hormonal fluctuations can affect the entire body, particularly the stomach.

Common Postmenopausal Changes

The many perimenopausal changes culminate in menopause. No more hot flashes! Most women heave a sigh of relief, because they believe the worst is now behind them. Unfortunately, however, that's not necessarily the case. The years following menopause bring their own particular set of challenges and changes. Many American women face new potential health risks. Again, each one of these problems can be resolved through the simple, safe, and effective natural remedies I'll outline later in the book. Here are some of the most common health problems that can afflict women in later life.

Osteoporosis

Osteoporosis is a condition that causes bones to become thin, brittle, and vulnerable to fracture. Bone tissue always breaks down, even in young and healthy individuals; in a healthy bone, however, new tissue is formed to replace the old tissue that has broken down. Degeneration is immediately followed by regeneration. This process is called bone resorption. For the bones to be able to regenerate, minerals such as calcium must be present. People with osteoporosis break down bone tissue faster than they can regenerate it, because the bones do not retain enough minerals and other important nutrients necessary to remain healthy and strong. These minerals are being leached from the bone and not replaced fast enough, or in sufficient quantities, due to dietary insufficiencies. Eventually, the skeleton weakens and becomes incapable of supporting daily activities. Some studies have linked osteoporosis to estrogen loss during the perimenopausal and menopausal period, because estrogen contributes to the ability of the bones to hold on to calcium.

Dental and Periodontal Changes

Many postmenopausal women experience a sharp decline in the health of their teeth and gums. The reason for this is the same as the reason for bone loss, and in fact, is closely related to osteoporosis. Since teeth are attached to the bone, bone loss will weaken the attachment of the teeth, and eventually allow them to fall out.

Of course, women who are in generally good dental health, and whose diet is low in sugar, are less likely to suffer from dental or periodontal disease; but every woman must, to some degree, be concerned with the condition of her teeth as she ages.

Cardiovascular Disease

Cardiovascular diseases affect the heart and circulatory system. Atherosclerosis (hardening of the arteries), hypertension (high blood pressure), angina, and stroke are among the most common manifestations. The number of American women who suffer from cardiovascular disease (CVD) is staggering. In fact, it is considered to be one of America's major killers. The physical changes that accompany menopause—particularly the drop in estrogen levels and the general aging of the blood vessels—set the stage for CVD and its insidious effects.

Urinary Incontinence

The lining of the urinary tract undergoes similar changes to those that take place in the lining of the vagina. It becomes thinner and less elastic with age. Occasionally, this makes women more susceptible to stress-related urinary incontinence. This condition does not mean that the incontinence is triggered by a fight with your boss or by a notification from the bank that your check bounced, but rather that it is brought on by physical activities—such as coughing, laughing, exercise, or lifting heavy objects—that might put pressure on the bladder. The presence of a urinary tract infection or a vaginal yeast infection further creates a predisposition to incontinence.

Coming to Terms with These Changes

If you have felt overwhelmed or frightened reading this list of changes that can take place during perimenopause and menopause, you are not alone. Sadly, all too many women in Western society continue to regard aging with horror and dread. While this consciousness is beginning to change, many women and many of their physicians continue to regard menopause as a disease rather than a natural and even beautiful process. What's interesting is that Asian women do not regard aging with the same distress as do their Western counterparts. Older women in Asia are venerated and respected as matriarchs and as wise community and family leaders. We can learn a great deal from these women, both physiologically and psychologically. We can learn about a diet that will curtail or even eliminate some of the most troublesome physiological menopausal symptoms. From a psychological point of view, we can learn just as much from their attitude to women and aging. Put simply, women are regarded as becoming more valuable as they age, and menopause is seen as a transition to a richer, more meaningful stage of life.

We will examine the Asian diet more extensively in chapter 3 and will focus on attitude and emotions in chapter 7. Suffice it to say here that you can join an increasing number of American women who are beginning to shift their attitude and embrace menopause as a positive process. A recent survey conducted by the Gallup Organization shows that more that half of the postmenopausal women interviewed reported feeling "happier and more fulfilled" than they were in their twenties. Many believed that they are better educated than their mothers and grandmothers and that they have access to better medical care and information. Most have utilized their knowledge to make important lifestyle changes, including alteration of nutritional habits, exercise, stress reduction, reduction in alcohol or nicotine consumption, and exploration of conventional or alternative approaches to hormonal health. The study showed that many of today's women are eager to reach out to younger women and assist them as they go through their own corridor of change.

This book can assist you in making those important lifestyle changes and reaching balanced and educated decisions regarding nutrition, exercise, and hormone replacement therapy. A positive and optimistic attitude will help to transform menopause from a dreaded experience, fraught with connotations of illness and decrepitude, to one of growth, change, and wonder.

Two

Hormone Replacement Therapy:
Pros and Cons

Let's talk about growing older. More to the point, let's talk about what it means to be a woman who is growing older.

In chapter 1, we discussed an array of physical and emotional experiences that most Western women go through during the menopausal years. Many of these bodily occurrences are a result of the aging process and affect men and women equally. As the body ages, its mechanisms tend to move more slowly and somewhat less efficiently. Think of your car. After a few years, your engine needs an adjustment. You need a brake job. Your directionals stop working or you need a new bulb in your headlight. What is true of cars is true of people as well. It is normal and it affects members of both genders.

My, that sounds grim, doesn't it? It really doesn't have to be. You can look and feel considerably younger than your years. Read on and you'll find out how—and particularly how you, as a woman, can utilize the *feminine* mechanisms of your body to age more youthfully. No, this is not a contradiction in terms—not when you understand how women age.

This chapter will explain how and why women age, and how conventional medicine has tried to address age-related health problems—such as cardiovascular disease, osteoporosis, and changes in sexual functioning—through hormone replacement therapy (HRT). We will examine this "treatment" carefully. We will look at whether it is effective, whether it is safe, and what other options might be available to you. Every woman must make a decision regarding HRT as she approaches her menopausal years. It is my hope that this chapter will provide you with some basic education regarding the complex issues involved in hormonal therapy. My aim is to inspire you to begin exploring safe, natural alternatives that will accomplish the same objectives as HRT, while simultaneously offering you assurances of safety and overall well-being that HRT does not provide.

Hormone Replacement Therapy

Everyone, whether male or female, experiences a series of changes as they move through middle age into the senior years. What affects women in particular are physical changes due to diminishing hormonal levels. The central hormones that play a role in the reproductive system are called "sex steroid hormones" and are the primary culprits in the menopausal changes. For example, many perimenopausal symptoms such as hot flashes, vaginal atrophy, headaches, and fatigue can be attributed to the sharp decrease in estrogen production by your ovaries. Even though estrogen is still produced by fat cells in your body, the amount is considerably smaller than what was previously secreted by your ovaries every month. Your entire body is affected by that change. Your body is also affected by changes in other sex steroid hormones, such as progesterone, testosterone, cortisol, and DHEA (dehydroepiandrosterone).

Many physicians today seek to boost diminishing estrogen levels through HRT. Let's have a brief look at how this method of treatment evolved, the forms in which it is offered, and the theory behind it.

The History of HRT

If you suffer from menopausal discomforts, you're certainly not alone. You and thousands of contemporary Western women are undergoing a similar set of experiences. You also have a great deal in common with your great-grandmothers and great-great-grandmothers. Indeed, menopausal difficulties have been described throughout history. For example, an eighteenth-century physician named John Leake wrote, "It may appear extraordinary that so many disorders should happen from a change so usual with every female."

It was unclear until the early twentieth century exactly what caused these menopausal "disorders." As scientific research progressed, the connection between estrogen and unpleasant menopausal symptoms was identified. Modern medicine sought to remedy these symptoms through estrogen replacement therapy (ERT), and then through hormone replacement therapy (HRT).

ERT was first attempted in the 1940s, when estrogen was given in large doses as a self-standing medication to women who were undergoing surgical menopause—that is, the removal of the ovaries and uterus. Women with intact ovaries and uteruses, however, were left to age unimpeded and unassisted by Western medicine until 1966. This is when the use of estrogen was popularized and brought into prominence with the publication of a book called *Feminine Forever,* by Robert A. Wilson, M.D. Women who read the book began to demand estrogen replacement therapy, believing that they would remain younger, healthier, and more attractive. An increasing number of doctors began to prescribe estrogen replacement therapy. In 1975, more than half the postmenopausal women—from 15 to 20 million of them—in the United States were using estrogen replacement therapy.

Social attitudes definitely contributed to the headlong rush of women to this apparent "fountain of youth." The medical establishment was only too glad to offer women "help" in forestalling the aging process and in calming their unpredictable female nerves. Perhaps this has something to do with the Western notion that we touched on in chapter 1—that only young women are beautiful and desirable, while older women are not. Doctors and their female patients collaborated in seeing aging as detrimental and youth-inducing treatments as desirable.

This attitude backfired. During the late 1970s, a disturbing series of reports linking estrogen replacement therapy to uterine cancer appeared. In fact, during the years when estrogen was being administered as a self-standing treatment, there was a 500 percent increase in uterine cancer! After an initial decline in the use of ERT, a new form of hormonal therapy was introduced. This modified hormonal therapy involved adding progestin (a synthetic form of progesterone) to the estrogen regimen in hopes of reducing the incidence of uterine cancer. The new, adjusted therapy—now called hormone replacement therapy (HRT)—is being used by millions of American women today. While there is still a substantial number of physicians who prescribe self-standing estrogen replacement therapy, most are now prescribing the newer modified hormone replacement combination. In fact, if you are a perimenopausal women complaining of hot flashes or irritability, it is likely that your gynecologist will whip out a prescription pad and prescribe HRT to you, promising that you will feel cool, calm, and collected.

What's the theory behind your doctor's claims? Let's understand why your doctor might believe that HRT is the solution to your problems.

Hormone Replacement Theory and Practice

Remember the menstrual cycle outlined in chapter 1? We described how your ovaries produce estrogen. Working together with progesterone, this is responsible for the regularity of the menstrual cycle. As you progress through your menopausal years, the production of estrogen and progesterone tapers off and almost stops. With this drop in hormonal levels comes menopause, with all its attendant discomforts.

The theory behind ERT, then, is a simple one. Estrogen is something essential to the healthy functioning of your body when you are young. Certain baseline levels of estrogen are necessary for the maintenance of regular and normal menstrual cycles. Estrogen contributes to bone and cardiac health, as well as vaginal lubrication and flexibility. It is known that diminished estrogen levels are responsible for some of the unpleasant physical and emotional effects of menopause, such as hot flashes, fatigue, irritability, and other discomforts. Physicians have therefore come to believe that replacing lost estrogen will maintain or even restore various "youthful" bodily functions.

Over the years, modern medicine has evolved several different forms of ERT. The most commonly prescribed estrogen replacement is administered orally through pills. These pills contain estrogen derived from the urine of pregnant mares. They are used because this form of estrogen is said to be similar in structure and function to human estrogens.

Estrogen replacement is also offered through adhesive patches, applied to the skin of the thigh or abdomen. The estrogen found in these patches is evenly and gradually absorbed through the skin, rather than through the gastrointestinal system. It is assumed that these patches result in fewer negative side effects because they are not ingested and because they contain less estrogen than do estrogen tablets.

There is also a somewhat less invasive form of estrogen therapy—estrogen creams. These creams are usually applied to the vaginal walls to provide the lubrication that is lost due to diminishing estrogen levels. They are prescribed particularly to women who suffer from vaginal atrophy or dryness. Although these creams are applied topically, they are absorbed systemically—that is, throughout the body.

It sounds as though ERT makes sense. But as you learned earlier in the chapter, the use of estrogen therapy alone causes as many problems as it solves. Remember the menstrual cycle? Estrogen predominates at the beginning of the cycle, as the uterine lining builds up in preparation for the possible advent of a fertilized egg. But progesterone predominates during the latter half of the cycle and is responsible for allowing the uterus to slough off its lining.

ERT provides the body with estrogen, which dutifully piles up the padding on the uterine walls. But without progesterone to balance out the process, the uterine walls simply keep getting thicker and thicker. The excessively thick uterine tissues are the perfect medium for the growth and proliferation of cancer cells.

For this reason, doctors have come up with hormone replacement therapy—an approach that combines estrogen with progestin. The progestin does what progesterone did during the menstrual cycle—it "instructs" the uterus to slough off its excess lining. This protects the uterus from being too padded and hospitable to cancer cells.

There are several different HRT regimens, each of which uses a different combination or sequence of estrogen and progestin. Some physicians prescribe estrogen from the first to the twenty-fifth day of each month and add a progestin tablet from the fourteenth to the twenty-fifth day. After day number twenty-five, the woman stops taking all hormones for five to six days. During that time, she may experience some bleeding, as if she were menstruating.

An alternative regimen involves taking a low-dose progestin pill together with estrogen throughout the month on a continuous basis. This eliminates the monthly periodlike effect of the first regimen. There is some intermittent and irregular spotting or staining at the beginning, but that usually clears up within six months to one year after starting the regimen.

Does that sound like the perfect solution? I wish it were. Sadly, while HRT solves many problems, it can cause many problems as well. The remainder of this chapter will help you evaluate HRT by examining its effectiveness in alleviating menopausal symptoms, its limitations and drawbacks, and the health risks with which it has been associated.

Does HRT Live Up to Its Claims?

If you are like many other women, your doctor might urge you to try HRT. In order to begin to make an informed decision regarding this course of action, you must ask yourself two important questions: What is HRT supposed to accomplish? And does it live up to its claims? This section will attempt to answer these questions by looking at each of the perimenopausal and postmenopausal problems that HRT is designed to relieve. In each case, we will examine how HRT is supposed to address the problem and whether scientific studies have actually substantiated the effectiveness of HRT.

Vaginal Atrophy or Dryness

As women age, their vaginal lining becomes dryer and less elastic, due to decreased levels of estrogen. This often leads to increased pain and discomfort, especially during intercourse. Estrogen replacement is said to rebuild the vaginal lining, provide lubrication, and increase resistance to friction.

HRT has indeed been demonstrated effective in dealing with vaginal atrophy and dryness, as well as the treatment of burning or difficult urination due to atrophy of the urethra or ureter. Numerous scientific studies suggest that HRT is helpful in improving the sex life of perimenopausal and postmenopausal women by creating a more hospitable vaginal climate.

Hot Flashes

Human beings are warm-blooded creatures. This means that our internal body temperature remains stable, despite any fluctuations and changes in climate and external temperature. (Reptiles and amphibians, for example, alter body temperature to conform to the temperature around them.) We are not lizards or frogs. Our bodies work hard to maintain their *homeostasis,* or sameness. If it is cold outside, we shiver, and the movement of our muscles keeps us warm by increasing the speed of blood flow and directing blood flow to the deeper body tissues. In hot weather, we sweat and flush. Sweat cools the body as it evaporates, and flushing brings more blood to the surface of the skin to be cooled.

Estrogen is an important component of this system. It helps the blood vessels in the skin to expand and contract, thereby regulating the consistency of body temperature. When estrogen levels drop, the system becomes less reliable. The sweating and flushing devices are not properly regulated, so routine stimuli that ordinarily would have no significant impact on the overall body temperature—hot drinks, caffeine, and stress, for instance—disrupt the balance. The body reacts as if it had been assaulted by a major heat wave. Many physicians believe that hot flashes are best addressed by replacing the lost estrogen through HRT. In fact, one of the most touted reasons for the use of HRT is its effectiveness in controlling hot flashes.

This claim is accurate. Reputable studies have confirmed that, most of the time, estrogen replacement therapy—with or without additional progestin—is successful in controlling hot flashes.

Cognitive Difficulties

Difficulties with memory or concentration are more troublesome to many women than are hot flashes. Most of my patients cite cognitive problems as being quite disruptive to their lives. The problems they encounter range from daily inconveniences, such as misplacing their keys or pocketbooks, to major problems, such as having trouble focusing on important tasks at work or at home. The same studies that supported the effectiveness of estrogen in controlling hot flashes have shown it does *not* remedy cognitive disturbances. Women using HRT experience the same lapses in memory and occasional episodes of disorientation and distractibility as do women who are not taking HRT.

Mood Disturbances

Anxiety, irritability, and depression are among the major presenting symptoms of many perimenopausal women. The symptoms are so pervasive that some misguided medical professionals prescribe antidepressants or sedatives to women whose primary complaints are mood related. Other physicians prescribe HRT because hormonal fluctuations are associated with disruptions in mood. (If you have ever suffered from PMS, you can attest to the significant impact of hormonal change upon your state of mind.)

Studies have failed to demonstrate that HRT has any positive impact on mood disturbances.

Loss of Libido

Estrogen, which is associated with youthfulness, is often thought to be the hormone responsible for the sexual drive. The frequent waning of libido during the perimenopausal and postmenopausal years is often attributed to diminishing levels of estrogen. HRT is supposed to remedy this situation.

Actually, estrogen is not the primary hormone involved in sexual arousal. Testosterone is the major hormone responsible for libido in women. Estrogen replacement has little, if any, value in the oft-stated complaint of low sex drive that afflicts many women before and after menopause.

Osteoporosis

I've already mentioned that in young women, estrogen is helpful in maintaining calcium levels in the bones. It is calcium that aids in the regeneration of bone tissue. When calcium is leached out of the bones, degeneration proceeds at a faster pace than regeneration, causing the bones to become brittle and fragile. The theory is that the estrogen introduced into the body through HRT will assist the bones in holding on to calcium, and thereby slow the degenerative process.

The current protocol, which combines HRT with some kind of calcium supplement, *does* appear to be effective in accomplishing this goal. Numerous studies have confirmed that HRT, begun immediately following menopause, is effective in combating osteoporosis. Most studies agree that women who are involved in an extended HRT regimen have 80 percent fewer hip fractures than their counterparts who are not taking HRT—*if* the treatment is continued for life. If the treatment is stopped, however, the bones degenerate at a much faster rate. (Scientists are still debating the effectiveness of HRT if it is initiated later in life—say, after age sixty. The current research indicates that it is probably ineffective in the prevention or treatment of osteoporosis.)

Cardiovascular Disease and Stroke

Estrogen has been linked with cardiac health. Studies have shown that it decreases the levels of "bad" cholesterol (LDL) in the blood while increasing levels of "good" (HDL) cholesterol. Since this cholesterol balance is so important to cardiac health, and since estrogen has also been shown to relax blood vessels and improve blood flow, it has been assumed that estrogen replacement will provide some protection against cardiovascular diseases such as atherosclerosis, angina, and stroke. In fact, cardiovascular benefits are among the most commonly stated reason doctors give in trying to convince apprehensive or skeptical women to start HRT treatment. This is a fact that never ceases to surprise me, because the results of the scientific studies are equivocal at best and many are actually quite negative. Some studies have implied that HRT has powerful cardiovascular benefits. Others challenge this notion. For example, a major study published in the August 1998 issue of the *Journal of the American Medical Association* showed that HRT did not decrease coronary heart disease in postmenopausal women. Many other studies have replicated and confirmed this finding.

Surgical Menopause

Women of reproductive age may undergo hysterectomies or oophorectomies (removal of the ovaries) because of repeated pelvic infections, cancer, fibroids, endometriosis, or hemorrhaging. This plunges them into what is called "surgical menopause." While they are chronologically youthful, their bodies are catapulted into the hormonal changes usually experienced by older women.

Hysterectomy and oophorectomy have a series of unpleasant aftereffects. If the ovaries have been removed, a sudden drop in hormone levels follows. The body must then adjust to a sudden and abrupt cessation of estrogen production, rather than the gradual changes of perimenopause. Most doctors prescribe HRT so as to stave off the depression, lack of sexual interest, fatigue, hot flashes, and vaginal atrophy that often follow the surgery.

Studies have shown that HRT is effective in that type of situation. Women who have undergone hysterectomy or oophorectomy do have an easier time if they are taking HRT. However, if organs have been removed because of cancer, conventional HRT is the last thing you should be considering! If hormone replacement therapy is required, the natural hormones described in chapter 7 will help you.

It is important for you to start on your program as soon as possible, because you do not have the luxury of time. Natural menopause happens gradually. You have time to incorporate new healthful behaviors into your life. Surgical menopause plunges your body into a dramatic estrogen short-age. It's a radical change, and requires focused and timely interventions.

My advice is that you work closely with a health-care provider in setting up your menopause program. You will need more support than the average woman going through menopause, because you have just undergone surgery—with all its attendant physical and emotional challenges—and because your need to create an effective program is immediate.

Does It Work or Not?

In answer to the question "Does HRT work?"—yes, it does work some of the time, for some of the problems. It *may* help with osteoporosis, vaginal atrophy and thinning, and hot flashes. It *does not* help with cardiovascular symptoms, fatigue, memory loss, irritability, loss of libido, or difficulty with concentration. It *does* alleviate most of the symptoms of surgical menopause.

At best we can say that HRT is a mixed blessing—or a mixed curse. Certainly, it can be helpful. But, as discussed earlier, it can also be harmful. And it has some additional major shortcomings. Despite what its supporters may tell you, HRT does not provide all the hormones you need to be at your best. And the hormones it does provide usually are not given to you in their most natural and helpful forms. The remainder of this chapter will examine each of these topics in turn. Finally—and most importantly—you will learn about naturally safe and effective alternatives to HRT. These accomplish the same goals without accompanying drawbacks and concerns.

What Are the Drawbacks of HRT?

HRT may be effective in addressing some perimenopausal problems—such as hot flashes—and some postmenopausal problems—such as osteoporosis—but its benefits come with a serious price tag.

The Missing Hormones

One of the drawbacks of HRT is that it may not replace all your missing or deficient hormones. HRT regimens are varied in nature but can be boiled down to two essential components—estrogen and progestin. But as we discussed earlier, your body actually produces five sex steroid hormones—estrogen, progesterone, testosterone, DHEA, and cortisol. Each of these hormones goes through fluctuations during the perimenopausal and postmenopausal years. The HRT regimens that are most commonly prescribed are based on guesswork. They are predicated on the assumption that women going through the menopausal transition are deficient in estrogen but that all the other hormones are present in normal levels.

While it is true that estrogen deficiency is more typical than deficiencies in other hormones, it is equally true that many women continue to have stable estrogen levels well into their senior years. Some women may even experience a rise in estrogen production as the ovaries go through their menopausal changes. But these women often are deficient in the other sex steroid hormones—testosterone, DHEA, or cortisol.

Low levels of testosterone can lead to symptoms such as fatigue, listlessness, and loss of libido. In fact, it is testosterone rather than estrogen deficiency that is most commonly responsible for the lack of sexual drive that many peri- and postmenopausal women experience. DHEA and cortisol are both associated with the body's ability to handle stress—to muster energy when a challenging situation arises, and to calm down when the crisis has passed. Women deficient in one or both of these hormones are often tired, while simultaneously feeling anxious and wound up. There have also been studies suggesting an association between DHEA levels and cognitive abilities. These studies imply that it is DHEA rather than estrogen that will assist menopausal women suffering from forgetfulness or distractibility.

A simple salivary test can accurately assess hormonal levels and pinpoint exactly which hormones are deficient, and which are excessive. Chapter 7 will teach you more about the salivary hormone test, as well as safe replacement of testosterone, DHEA, and cortisol.

Estrogen—It's Not As Simple As You Think

Throughout this chapter, we have been referring to "estrogen" as if it were a single substance. Actually, there are three different types of estrogen—estradiol, estrone, and estriol—and each has its own particular function.

The estrogen that is secreted by the ovaries is called *estradiol*. It is the most potent of the three and is the estrogen that predominates during the premenopausal, reproductive years. During the childbearing years, it is estradiol that travels to the breasts, assists with lactation, and builds the uterine lining in preparation for the baby. Estradiol binds to receptor sites in the bones to keep them young and healthy; binds to sites in the vagina to keep the vaginal walls moist, supple, and elastic; and travels through the bloodstream, promoting cardiovascular health. But during the menopausal years, estriol predominates. An excess of estradiol during those years is harmful. The body of a postmenopausal woman should convert estradiol into estrone and, in turn, into estriol. When all the appropriate biochemical substances are present in the gastrointestinal tract and liver, the body accomplishes this conversion process efficiently, and there is little if any free-floating estradiol in the body. The estrogen now present is estriol. It exercises the same beneficial effect on the vaginal lining and cardiovascular system but is an estrogen specifically suited to the postmenopausal system.

If you lack the appropriate enzymes and other substances in your gut and liver, you may not properly convert estradiol into estriol, and you may have an overabundance of estradiol in your body. This particular form of estrogen—once so essential to the reproductive functions of your body—actually becomes a carcinogen once you have concluded the childbearing chapter of your life. An overabundance of free-floating estradiol in a woman's body often leads to cancer, and particularly to breast cancer. The reason for this is that the breasts contain *estrogen receptors*. These are sites that are biochemically constructed so as to attract free-floating estrogens. During your reproductive years, estradiol is important for maintaining breasts that can nurse a baby. The estrogen receptors are seeking this particular variety of estrogen, and receiving it does not lead to disease. After menopause, however, the entire hormonal environment changes. When the postmenopausal body is functioning with good health, and the balance between estradiol and estriol is correct (low estradiol levels and high estriol levels), then the estriol that binds to breast receptors protects the breasts from cancer. When the reverse is the case—estradiol levels are high and estriol levels are low—then the unhealthy estrogen binds to receptor sites in the breast and can lead to breast cancer.

For reasons that I cannot understand, most American HRT (in contrast to European HRT) consists of estradiol rather than estriol or estrone. The large quantity of free-floating estradiol introduced into the body binds to estrogen receptors in the breast. Estradiol "fools" the breast receptors into regarding it as a "friend" instead of an enemy, often leading to breast cancer.

Studies have shown that European postmenopausal women receiving hormone treatment have a lower incidence of breast cancer than do their American counterparts. This is largely due to the type of estrogen that European women receive. We will return to this subject in chapter 7, when we look at safe and natural hormone replacement options.

Horses, Chemicals, and Human Beings

The estrogen used in American HRT is taken, as I mentioned above, from the urine of pregnant mares. I'm not a horse. You're not a horse. We have human, not equine, bodies. Animal-based estrogen may be somewhat similar, but is not identical to, human estrogen. It works quite differently in the human body.

Estrogen isn't the only problem. The progesterone used in HRT is equally problematic, because it is not identical to the progesterone that our body actually makes. It's called progestin, and it's a synthetic imitation of the real McCoy. It just doesn't work the way authentic progesterone works. Even real progesterone has its serious drawbacks, as we'll see below. The problem with progestin is that it has all the disadvantages of progesterone, plus a host of its own unique disadvantages. Progestin exaggerates and multiplies the unpleasant effects of progesterone, to the point of actual risk.

Keep these introductory comments in mind while we look at the problems that have been associated with HRT.

Health Risks Associated With HRT

Studies have associated HRT with an array of medical conditions. Some of these are very serious indeed. Others—while less alarming—are nevertheless annoying, affecting the quality of life. Here are some of the health risks posed by all forms of conventional American HRT—oral pills, patches, and creams.

Cancer   While the incidence of uterine cancer *has* dropped from the 500 percent increase that occurred when ERT was first introduced, the fact is that we still see a 30 percent increase in uterine cancer in women

Discontinuing HRT If You've Already Started

Many of my patients, concerned about the negative effects of HRT, ask me if it's safe to discontinue hormone replacement in favor of the more natural approaches outlined in this book. I assure them that it's safe and completely desirable—but I advise them to do so under medical guidance, rather than independently.

If you are currently taking estrogen and wish to discontinue your treatments, my advice is that you work with your health-care provider—especially if you have been using estrogen for an extended period of time. With careful monitoring of your hormonal levels, you should be able to taper off your HRT treatments as you begin incorporating the suggestions in this book into your lifestyle.

Your physician may also wish to assess your bone mineral density. Since discontinuation of ERT places a woman at somewhat higher risk for developing osteoporosis, you should place special emphasis on following the recommendations in this book for building healthy bones.

using HRT, as compared with women who are not taking hormones at all. Studies have linked estrogen-progestin compounds with breast and ovarian cancer. In 1997, the British medical journal *Lancet* reported that fifty-one studies conducted in twenty-one countries, with a total of 53,865 postmenopausal participants using HRT, showed a risk of breast cancer that increased by 1 percent for every year of HRT use. In 1999, researchers published the results of the Iowa Women's Health Study in the *Journal of the American Medical Association*. A multi-university group of scientists followed 37,105 postmenopausal women over an eleven-year period. They concluded that exposure to HRT was strongly associated with a risk of invasive breast cancer. As this book was going to press, another crucial study was published. It confirmed, once again, that estrogen replacement therapy significantly increases the risk of breast cancer. Researchers at the National Cancer Institute studied 46,355 women at twenty-nine breast cancer screening centers in the United States over a four-year period. They studied the potential cancer-causing effects of commonly prescribed estrogen and estrogen-progestin combination therapy in postmenopausal women. The study, which was published in the January 26, 2000, issue of the *Journal of the American Medical Association,* showed that the risk of breast cancer increased with each form of therapy for each year of use. At the end of the four-year study period, the researchers concluded that estrogen replacement increased the risk of breast cancer by approximately 20 percent. Estrogen-progestin replacement increased the risk of breast cancer by approximately 40 percent of those women who were on hormonal therapy during the study period. Many other studies have replicated this finding. Also, as mentioned above, while HRT reduces the risk of uterine cancer associated with the use of estrogen, it by no means eliminates that risk.

Cardiovascular Problems   HRT has been associated with increased risk of high blood pressure, cardiovascular disease, and stroke. HRT has also been linked with an increased incidence of thromboembolism (blood clots in the veins)—a very serious and potentially life-threatening condition. The August 1999 study referred to above, published in the *Journal of the American Medical Association,* concluded that there is "no overall cardiovascular benefit [to HRT] and there is a pattern of early increase in the risk of coronary heart disease." That finding has been replicated in several other major studies.

PMS-like Symptoms   Progesterone is what gives you the "yucky" feeling that so many women complain about during the days immediately before the onset of your menstrual period. Progesterone is implicated in the irritability, fatigue, breast tenderness, abdominal discomfort, and other unpleasant symptoms of PMS. Women who take progestin on a consistent basis—and even those who take it for a few weeks each month and then stop—feel that they have PMS all the time. Many studies have shown that HRT contributes to breast tenderness and discomfort. The very reason for embarking upon a course of hormonal therapy—to alleviate unpleasant sensations associated with menopause—ends up being defeated. You may not experience hot flashes and night sweats, but you are still irritable, tired, bloated, and uncomfortable in your breast area. So just as you're kissing your PMS symptoms good-bye, there they are again! This, too, is a frying-pan-and-fire effect.

Uterine Fibroids   HRT has been associated with an increase in uterine fibroids—benign overgrowths of muscular uterus tissue. These growths enlarge the uterus and can be quite painful. At their worst, they must be surgically removed, although there are other ways to handle some fibroids.

The estrogen in HRT, which causes growth of the uterine lining, also stimulates the growth of fibroids. Even progestin does not balance out this effect. Women who have suffered from fibroids should be able to look forward to relief after menopause, when estrogen levels diminish; but HRT can cause the fibroids to keep growing, and relief may come only through surgery.

Other Discomforts   HRT can lead to fluid retention, weight gain, and increased susceptibility to yeast infections. Most women are never warned of these risks, nor are they advised to discontinue HRT if they have begun to experience chronic yeast infections. HRT has also been associated with vaginal bleeding, skin problems such as acne, and alterations in mood, such as anxiety or depression. Again, these symptoms are caused by progestin.

Noncompliance   Some physicians complain that there is a high noncompliance rate with HRT. In other words, many women do not follow the prescribed regimen. These women find that progestins make them feel worse than estrogen alone, and simply stop taking the progestin. This can be quite dangerous because of the risk of uterine cancer posed by taking estrogen alone.

By now I'm sure you'll agree that this is quite a laundry list of problems associated with an ostensible solution!

A Natural Approach to Menopause and Aging

The remainder of this book will focus on effective and risk-free solutions to your menopausal problems. For example, diet—discussed in chapter 3—provides natural hormone replacement. Aside from nutrients such as vitamins and minerals that contribute to general good health, your diet can provide nutrients that specifically contribute to menopausal wellness and hormonal balance. These nutrients, called *phytoestrogens,* are present in soy products and garbanzo beans, and in many fruits and vegetables.

An array of powerful vitamins, minerals, herbs, homeopathic remedies, and other nutritional supplements can help you to cope with the full range of menopausal symptoms. Chapter 4 will provide you with a detailed list of these supplements, and how to use them.

Chapter 5 will teach you how to use exercise—an invigorating and safe activity—to feel better in general, and to combat many common perimenopausal and postmenopausal problems—particularly cardiovascular disease and osteoporosis.

If you feel you want additional hormonal support during this time, you can turn to chapter 7. It will suggest safer—and often more natural—hormones that your doctor can prescribe. These hormones will directly address your own personal profile of hormonal imbalances and deficiencies, and will rectify them in a highly focused, safe, and rigorous fashion. They will help you move gently through the processes of menopause and aging.

The word *aging* brings us back full circle to the image of the car. Your car may change with age, but if you give it regular tune-ups and keep the oil changed and the transmission fluid up to date, these problems take much longer to manifest, and are much more easily resolved. The same is true of your health. Your organs and cells do undergo some degeneration as you age; but with a healthy lifestyle, you can slow down many of the changes and so-called negative experiences associated with this delicate time.

We've established that you're not a lizard or frog, and that you're not a horse. You are also not a car. A car is a machine, lacking consciousness and consisting only of its mechanical parts. You are a human being with thoughts, feelings, and beliefs, and your attitude and sense of personal empowerment will have a dramatic impact on your health. Taking a proactive approach to hormone replacement and incorporating natural alternatives into your lifestyle will give your body the gift of health-building, natural, and effective aids to vibrant aging.

Three

Diet: Your Best Hormone Replacement Therapy

Time to keep my promise. In chapter 2, I warned you about the hazards of HRT. I told you that there are safer and equally effective measures to address your perimenopausal and postmenopausal concerns. This chapter is devoted to the first of these measures—diet. A well-balanced diet is essential to good health at all stages of life, and particularly during the menopausal years.

In this chapter, you will learn about phytohormones—the substances in soybeans, chickpeas, and vegetables that have been found to be so effective in combating a variety of menopause-related symptoms and disorders. Then you will learn how a generally well-balanced diet can be equally important in helping you maintain health during menopause. You will discover that some foods, such as whole grains, can help you look and feel your best; while other foods, such as red meats and refined sugars, can compromise your health. Finally, some simple guidelines for good eating will help you put these principles into practice so that you can easily create a diet that meets your nutritional needs now and for the rest of your life.

Phytonutrients—The Key to Menopausal Health

I'm sure you are aware that a well-balanced diet is essential to building and maintaining good health. I'm also sure that you are familiar with the names of many necessary components of the foods you eat. For example, most of you probably know that vitamins and minerals are crucial to good health.

You are probably aware that oranges contain vitamin C, which is helpful in preventing and fighting colds. But there are food components I bet you've never heard of. For example, did you ever hear of eating broccoli because it is a rich source of indoles? How about eating an apple because it is a rich source of flavonoids? These other plant compounds—known as *phytonutrients*—are as important to your health as the vitamins and minerals you learned about when you were a child. In fact, the study of phytonutrients is at the cutting edge of modern scientific research.

Phytonutrients are nonvitamin, nonmineral plant compounds. Many prevent cancer and heart disease, while others protect the liver against toxic insult. Still others help keep bones healthy and strong. You'd be amazed at how healthful they really are, and how many studies support their effectiveness! Vegetables, for example, contain anticarcinogenic substances. These include antioxidant vitamins such as carotenoids, vitamin C, vitamin E, antioxidant minerals such as selenium, and phytonutrients such as isoflavones, dithiolthiones, isothiocyanates, indoles, phenols, and protease inhibitors. And if that's not enough, vegetables contain a host of other protective substances, many of which scientists haven't even begun to explore yet.

Numerous studies have shown that people who consume more vegetables, fruits, whole grains, and legumes have a generally lower risk of contracting all kinds of cancer—colon, rectum, breast, uterus, and stomach—to name just a few. Women who eat large quantities of these wholesome foods also have a more balanced hormonal system, especially during the menopausal years. Vegetables and soybeans are cheaper and safer than estrogen tablets. (They're also a lot more tasty and enjoyable!) In the next section, we will take a closer look at the phytonutrients present in vegetables, fruits, and legumes and the role they can play in your menopausal program. These *phytohormones*—plant hormones—can actually provide a viable alternative to hormone replacement therapy.

"Eat Your Vegetables, Dear, and Your Soybeans Too"

Remember when Mom urged you to eat your vegetables? I bet she didn't say, "Because vegetables contain phytohormones that will prevent hot flashes when you're a grown-up." Or "One day you will want to protect yourself against breast cancer." And I imagine she didn't tout the virtues of soybeans or legumes either, probably because she wasn't aware of these things. Soybeans are not an integral part of the Western diet, and their connection to hot flashes and other menopausal phenomena are only now becoming understood by the scientific community.

Scientists began investigating phytohormones when they began to realize that Asian women do not experience hot flashes and other physical discomforts associated with the pre- and postmenopausal years. Nor do they suffer from as much breast cancer as we do in this country. But second- and third-generation Asian women living in the United States who have adopted the American lifestyle and diet have a risk of breast cancer and hot flashes equivalent to that of American women.

As scientists thoroughly studied the lifestyle of Asian women, they realized that the Asian diet is vastly different from the Western diet in one significant respect—Asian women eat considerably more vegetables than do their Western counterparts. They also consume larger quantities of soy. In fact, one of the staples of the Asian diet is tofu, or soybean curd. Scientists who studied soybeans began to realize that these Asian staples are rich in phytohormones, or plant hormones. They theorized that these plant hormones were supplying, through dietary means, what HRT was supplying through pharmacological means. They studied vegetables and theorized that vegetables, too, contain substances that have an estrogen-like impact on the body.

These "theories" have been borne out by extensive scientific study in recent years. The phytohormones in soy and vegetables definitely mitigate many menopausal discomforts, such as hot flashes, and do appear to prevent more serious conditions, such as breast cancer. Let's look at how this works.

How Phytoestrogens Work in the Body

Phytoestrogens serve multiple purposes. To begin with, they are similar to estriol—the form of estrogen most desirable during the postmenopausal years—in their structure. This structural similarity enables the phytoestrogens to mimic the effect of estriol in the body. They bind to estrogen receptor sites in the breast and serve as protection against free-floating estradiol (the form of estrogen least desirable during the postmenopausal years). They also protect the breasts from the insidious invasion of *xenoestrogens*. These estrogenlike substances are found in chemical pesticides such as DDT, in pollutants, in the breakdown of plastics, and in other toxic substances. Because xenoestrogens are so similar to estrogen, they bind to estrogen receptor sites in the breasts and elsewhere, and become carcinogenic.

People who consume large quantities of phytoestrogens keep those receptor sites busy with healthy, protective substances. The estriol-like phytohormones bind to the receptor sites, rendering them unavailable for the invading xenoestrogens, and also for any free-floating estradiol that the liver has not managed to convert into estriol. There's an old saying: "The devil finds work for idle hands to do." When estrogen receptors in the breasts and in other parts of the body are "idle," they are more vulnerable to the evil workings of the "devil"—the xenoestrogen or estradiol cell that hooks up to the receptor site, leading to breast cancer.

An equally important function of phytoestrogens is in the actual conversion of estradiol into estriol. The liver uses phytoestrogens extensively in its conversion process. Phytoestrogens facilitate the healthy functioning of the liver, and therefore increase the amount of estriol in the body.

So we see that phytoestrogens are very important. In their own right, they provide the body with enough estrogenlike substances that the health of the bones, the vaginal lining, and the cardiovascular system are augmented. Bodily occurrences linked with low estrogen levels—such as hot flashes—are greatly reduced or even eliminated, because the body is taking in a substance that mimics the effect of healthy estrogen. Breast health is protected, because phytoestrogens provide safe and healthy substances to shield the breast from dangerous imposters, or from elevated estradiol levels. Last, phytoestrogens facilitate the conversion of estradiol into estriol, and restore a healthy balance between the two.

Can Phytoestrogens Replace HRT?

They certainly can. Used correctly, phytoestrogens render HRT unnecessary. The research regarding phytoestrogens has resoundingly supported seeing them as viable alternatives to HRT. Study after study has demonstrated their effectiveness, and also their safety.

Unfortunately, some physicians who might be open to incorporating the use of phytoestrogens into their practice are hesitant because they do not believe that it is realistic. One well-known gynecologist, affiliated with a major teaching hospital, expressed this succinctly: "I'm sure the stuff works, and it's a nice idea in theory. But American women are different from Asian women. It's just not realistic to expect American women to eat pounds and pounds of soybeans every day, and to live on vegetables all the time. American women also don't want to alter their eating habits. It's easier for them to just swallow a pill."

This doctor is wrong! It is not unrealistic, or terribly complicated, to evolve a lifestyle that incorporates regular and effective quantities of phytoestrogens into the diet. You don't need to shovel voluminous quantities of soybeans into your mouth. Even a serving a day of a food that is rich in phytoestrogens—such as soybeans or chickpeas—as well as some of the phytonutrient-rich cruciferous vegetables—those plants in the cabbage family, such as Brussels sprouts, broccoli, kale, and cauliflower—will go a long way toward improving your hormonal health. Table 3:1 will provide a sampling of a few important sources of phytoestrogens, and will show you how much of each food constitutes a serving.

It is important to vary your intake of phytoestrogen-containing foods. Soy products are the most well-known source of phytoestrogens. They contain *isoflavones*—an important phytoestrogen indeed. There are other types of phytoestrogens, however. *Lignans,* for example, are found in legumes, whole grains, cruciferous vegetables, and flaxseeds. Flaxseeds are by far the most concentrated source of lignans, and can be incorporated into your diet in a variety of interesting ways.

"Interesting" is the key here. You don't have to sit down to a grim meal of unadorned soybeans in order to have a diet rich in phytoestrogens. A veggie burger sandwich, for example, is a delicious and excellent source of varied phytoestrogens. The burger might contain soy protein as well as chopped vegetables, such as carrots, onions, garlic, and celery. Garnishing your whole-grain sandwich with lettuce and tomatoes adds different phytonutrients, as well as color and flavor. Salads, chickpea spreads, and stir-fried vegetables with tofu are all interesting and tasty sources of phytoestrogens. Soymilk can be added to hot or cold cereal and can be used in baking as a substitute for milk. Because tofu is a tasteless substance, it "disappears" into other foods and takes on their flavor. You can add it to casseroles, salads, and stews. You can sprinkle flaxseeds on salads or cereals, or blend them into fruit shakes. They taste slightly nutty, and add a wonderful and unusual flavor to all your dishes. Kudzu, beans, and lentils all contain some phytohormones and can be used in a variety of interesting ways.

There are also safe and natural nutritional supplements that contain phytoestrogens. Chapter 4 will provide you with detailed guidelines to natural phytoestrogen supplementation.

Table 3:1 Servings of Phytoestrogen-Rich Foods

Soybeans and Garbanzo Beans	
Soybeans (cooked)	1/2 cup
Garbanzo beans (cooked)	1/2 cup
Humus	1/2 cup
Tofu	4–6 oz
Soy milk	6–8 oz
Textured soy protein (TVP)	1/4 cup dry
Miso	2 tablespoons
Miso soup	1 cup
Soy flour	1/4 cup
Soy hot dog	2 hot dogs
Soy nuts	1/4 cup
Tofu yogurt	1 cup
Cruciferous Vegetables	
Broccoli	1 cup
Kale	1 cup
Cabbage	1 cup
Brussels sprouts	1 cup
Cauliflower	1 cup
Watercress	1 cup
Radishes	1 cup
Collard greens	1 cup

The Building Blocks of a Healthy Diet

Did you learn about "basic food groups" when you were young? I remember sitting in health class as my home-economics teacher pointed a ruler at pictures of steak, butter, white bread, and apple pie. Today's scientists have discovered that these types of food may be injurious rather than beneficial to health. They have learned that there are really four major *nutrients* that are the building blocks of a healthy diet: fat, proteins, complex carbohydrates, and water. You also need micronutrients—vitamins and minerals—which are no less essential to good health, but are needed in considerably smaller quantities.

The major nutrients of your diet should be eaten in proportions that are somewhat different from what your home-economics teacher might have believed. Modern nutritionists recommend that 60 percent of your daily food intake consist of complex, unrefined carbohydrates, 20 percent of protein, and only 20 percent of fat. By "fat" I don't mean egg yolks, chopped liver, or ice cream. I am talking about monounsaturated un-heated oils such as extra-virgin olive oil or the oils naturally provided in whole foods such as nuts, avocados, and certain vegetables. Additionally, your diet should provide 25 grams of fiber—something that your home-economics teacher or school nurse might have called "roughage"—and approximately eight glasses of water. Let's look at each of these.

Fats

As a clinical nutritionist, I am always surprised by how much confusion my patients express concerning the subject of fat and how much misin-formation abounds in our culture. We all know that eating too much fat can make us fat. In our weight-conscious society, most of us are aware of how important it is to lower our fat intake in order to lower our weight. Most of us are also aware of the connection between fat consumption and heart disease, and hardly a day goes by without some news report of a study linking fat consumption to cancer.

When we hear the word *fat,* then, we think of a single type of food. In truth, there are many different types of fat. Some should be avoided, while others should be eaten in specific quantities and proportions. I'd like to clarify which types of fat are beneficial to your health, which are detrimental, and why.

Saturated and Polyunsaturated Fats   We have been warned by the American Heart Association that too much saturated fat—the kind found in red meat, hard cheese, butter, and egg yolks—builds layers of plaque along the arteries, leading to atherosclerosis, or hardening of the arteries. This condition, in turn, leads to heart attacks and strokes. In response to this concern, many Americans switched from butter to margarine, and to "lite" fat products, such as reduced-fat mayonnaise and salad dressings. These products contain polyunsaturated fats, which were at one time touted as a solution to heart disease.

Today's scientists know that this is a mistaken approach. Large quantities of polyunsaturated fats—which are found in nuts, seeds, sunflower, safflower, and corn oils—actually contribute to the aging process by adding chemicals called free radicals to your bloodstream. These damaging substances attack the cell structure in your body, causing a process called oxidation to occur. In small quantities, this is a normal process and will not be harmful. An excess of free radicals, however, has been associated with disorders such as arthritis, cancer, and cardiovascular disease, and with visual and mental degeneration. Even eating large quantities of vegetables and fruits containing antioxidant vitamins such as vitamin E, vitamin C, and beta-carotene will not always counteract the detrimental effects of the avalanche of free radicals produced by the polyunsaturated fats that abound in our American diet. Small quantities of these fats are harmless and even contain ingredients necessary for good health, but large quantities contribute to the very illnesses that they were supposed to mitigate.

Hydrogenated oils, too, were once considered to be a safe alternative to butter and high-cholesterol vegetable oils, such as coconut oil. Hydrogenation involves adding hydrogen to liquid vegetable oil in order to form solid margarine or shortening. Again, modern research has shown that hydrogenated oils are not viable alternatives to saturated fats, because they produce trans-fatty acids in the body. These trans-fatty acids act in much the way that saturated fat does. They raise blood cholesterol levels and may even be linked to some kinds of cancer.

It is especially important to avoid saturated and hydrogenated fats during the perimenopausal and postmenopausal years because they build fat cells in the body. Those fat cells produce and release estradiol into the system. As you learned in chapter 2, estradiol—an estrogen produced in abundance during the reproductive years—is destructive to the body during the postreproductive years. It binds to estrogen receptor sites in the breast, building up breast tissue and increasing the risk of breast cancer. In fact, study after study has demonstrated that reducing fat intake reduces the risk of breast cancer.

Does that mean that fat should be completely eliminated from your diet? Do you always have to push away the succulent steak, the crisp french fries, or the frosty milk shake? Not at all. You can safely enjoy small quantities of these foods on occasion, rather than large quantities on a daily basis. No one has ever become obese from indulging in a rich dessert once a week. The key is once a week! It is the daily coffee-with-cream-and-danish breakfast, rather than the occasional splurge, that is the problem. Your guiding principle should be to make the consumption of saturated, polyunsaturated, and hydrogenated fats the rare exception, rather than the rule.

You do need some polyunsaturated fats. We will discuss them more extensively in the section below.

Essential Fatty Acids   It may surprise you to learn that there is a kind of fat that should be added to your diet. Perhaps your mother grew up grimacing as her mother or grandmother poured a tablespoon of cod-liver oil into her mouth. Mine certainly did. Cod-liver oil may have tasted awful, but it had its benefits. Our ancestors had some awareness that fish oil is beneficial to health. Mom was sometimes very wise, and so was Grandma.

This old-fashioned notion has been revived and confirmed by modern science. Scientists noticed that Eskimos do not suffer from cancer or heart disease, even though they consume large quantities of whale blubber. The scientists realized that the fish oil, which constitutes a staple of the Eskimo diet, protects against cardiovascular disease, cancer, asthma, and arthritis.

Why is fish oil so beneficial to your health? Fish oil belongs to a category of fats that are actually needed for good health. Called essential fatty acids (EFAs), these fats cannot be manufactured by our bodies, and so they must be provided by our diets. The two most important groups of EFAs are the omega-3 and the omega-6 fatty acids.

You will find omega-3 fatty acids in cold-water fish and seafood, such as herring, salmon, tuna, cod, mackerel, and shrimp, in flaxseeds and flaxseed oils, and in some leafy green plant foods. These fats include several substances essential to your health—alpha-linolenic acid, eicosapentaenoic acid (EPA), and docosahexaenoic acid (DHA). Your body metabolizes alpha-linolenic acid by turning it into EPA and finally into DHA. DHA is the end product, the form most usable by your body. This is the substance that your body uses to accomplish a variety of important functions, such as fighting inflammation, cancer, and heart disease. While all the foods mentioned above contain omega-3 fatty acids, only fish oils contain preformed EPA and DHA. By eating fish, you save your body a few steps and give it the compounds it most needs in ready-made form.

Most Americans eat considerably more omega-6 than omega-3 foods. These are found in certain plants and vegetable oils—such as corn, sunflower, safflower, and canola. The omega-6 family includes cis-linoleic acid, linoleic acid, and gamma-linolenic acid (GLA). We rarely consume foods high in GLA, the most therapeutic form of the omega-6 family. (After all, how many of us regularly eat foods with evening primrose, borage, or black currant oils?) Most of us also do not consume enough of the omega-3 group to counterbalance our large intake of omega-6 foods. Scientists estimate that our ancestors probably consumed a diet consisting of an equal balance of omega-3 and omega-6 fatty acids. All that changed, however, with the Industrial Revolution, when cultural and technological factors led to altered eating habits. People ate more fatty meats and diets higher in vegetable oils. The formerly equal balance of fatty acids became dramatically lopsided, as Westerners began to consume twenty times more omega-6 than omega-3 foods.

An imbalance in fatty acids is problematic, because all these substances are eventually converted by the body into prostaglandins. These are hormonelike substances produced and used by our cells. Once manufactured, the prostaglandins regulate all bodily functions, including those of the cardiovascular, reproductive, immune, and nervous systems. Prostaglandins have several different effects, all of which are necessary. Interestingly, they can accomplish two apparently contradictory ends, depending on what the body needs at any given time. For example, prostaglandins can have anti-inflammatory as well as pro-inflammatory effects. The balance between the two depends on achieving the correct dietary balance between the two kinds of EFAs.

Working together, EFAs are very powerful. They serve as structural parts of the cell membranes in our bodies and therefore help protect our cells from invading toxins, bacteria, viruses, carcinogens, and allergens. It's easy to understand why research has linked fatty acid imbalances to a variety of chronic diseases, including cardiovascular disease, arthritis, allergies, and an array of immunological disorders.

During the reproductive years, a correct balance in EFAs will help reduce symptoms of premenstrual syndrome (PMS), such as depression and irritability, as well as the cramps, nausea, bloating, and headaches associated with dysmenorrhea—painful menstrual periods. Studies have shown that women who experience difficult PMS each month are more likely to have the same or similar set of experiences during perimenopause. Rectifying EFA imbalances will help modulate the hormonal imbalances responsible for such symptoms as hot flashes, irritability, depression, headaches, gastrointestinal disturbances, and breast tenderness.

For postmenopausal women, cardiovascular disease is one of the most central concerns—and also one of the most common reasons many physicians encourage the use of HRT, believing that the estrogen will help protect against heart attacks and strokes. Studies show that some of the substances in EFAs—specifically EPA, DHA, and GLA—protect against heart disease. Platelets—the blood cells that enable our blood to clot and aggregate—can adhere to artery walls, contributing to atherosclerosis. By preventing this adhesion, EFAs act as natural "blood thinners" that are far safer than the aspirin treatment often prescribed by doctors for this purpose. EFAs are not associated with the ulcers, gastrointestinal bleeding, anemia, and other side effects that occur with aspirin use. In studies that used both aspirin and fish oil, for example, the combination was more effective than aspirin alone. EFAs also appear to lower high levels of triglycerides—a risk factor in heart disease.

Studies have even suggested that EFAs are effective in the treatment of existing heart disease. There is evidence that fish oil, for example, lowers blood pressure and can reduce chest pain during exercise in people with angina. Because of its blood-thinning abilities, EPA may also be of use after bypass surgery and as an adjunct to angioplasty. In addition, GLA has been shown to reduce stress-induced hypertension in animals, and to help relieve the pain of angina in human beings.

Fish oil is probably the easiest EFA to incorporate into your diet, because all you have to do is switch from a meat-centered diet to a fish-centered diet. This is not a very complicated task at all. You don't even have to eat fish every day! Just try adding salmon to your menu a couple of times a week. If you don't like fish, however, you can use other foods containing EFAs.

While EPA and DHA can easily be incorporated into your diet by eating seafood or fish—specifically fatty fish, like tuna fish or salmon—at least three times a week, it is difficult to get a sufficient amount of GLA just from food. Some commercial oils such as canola, for example, contain GLA, but most contain linoleic acid. For this reason, I generally recommend EFA supplementation, especially for those with cholesterol levels above 180. Chapter 4 will discuss the supplements and quantities.

Supplementation is probably a good idea for everyone, even those whose cholesterol levels are low. Eating foods rich in EFAs is important, but it may not be enough. The conversion process in which the body must engage to take the alpha-linolenic acid found in, say, flaxseed oil and convert it into EPA and DHA, or to take the linoleic acid found in canola oil and convert it into GLA, is often impeded by other dietary and lifestyle factors. These include smoking, environmental toxins, aging, excessive saturated fat intake, alcohol, sugar, and stress. We will discuss this at greater length in chapter 4.

Protein

Protein—which should comprise 20 percent of your daily calories—is made up of amino acids. These essential building blocks of our health must be supplied through our diet, because our bodies cannot manufacture them. Amino acids are necessary for maintaining healthy bones, skin, hormones, muscle tissue, and neurotransmitters.

I've noticed that many of my patients are confused about protein. Some, who are trying to reduce cholesterol, have eliminated meat, chicken, and dairy from their diet without substituting any healthier form of protein. They are surprised that they feel weak, crave sweets, and are hungry all the time. Other patients eat an excess of protein, believing this will build healthy bones, muscles, and teeth. They do not realize that diets too high in protein can cause calcium to be lost from the body, contributing to osteoporosis, and that high-protein diets also place an extra burden on the kidneys, which must work extra hard to break down any excess protein the body can't use. Many of these people eat so much protein at a meal that they have no room for essential foods such as vegetables, fruits, and whole grains, so they lose out on the wide range of phytonutrients necessary for maintaining good health. (Indeed, our American diet is constructed around protein as the center of a meal, and vegetables as "side dishes.")

Finally, a high-protein diet often consists of foods high in cholesterol—such as red meat—which is known to contribute to cardiovascular disease.

As with so many other aspects of healthy eating, the key to proper protein consumption lies in balance and moderation—and in choosing proteins that are most beneficial to your health. So while animal products—including fish, eggs, milk, meat, and chicken—provide all the eight essential amino acids, soy might be a better choice of protein because it is low in cholesterol and extremely high in phytoestrogens. It's true that animal products constitute the most common source of protein in the Western diet. However, there are many people in different parts of the world who do not eat a Western diet. Asians, for example, use meat and chicken as a condiment or side dish—exactly the reverse of how we use these animal products in the United States. Specifically, much of the protein that Asian people consume comes from soybeans and fish, which is probably the main reason why Asian women do not have some of the perimenopausal and postmenopausal discomforts and ailments that plague most Western women.

It is especially important for women to avoid large quantities of red meat, poultry, and dairy products during their menopausal years because these products contain hormones that are fed to livestock to promote their growth as well as xenoestrogens contained in the pesticides sprayed on animal feed. These hormones and xenoestrogens can bind to estrogen receptors in the breast, increasing the risk of breast cancer. Meat, poultry, eggs, and dairy also contain antibiotics, which the animals are given so that they remain healthy in extremely cramped quarters.

All these substances are quite toxic to human beings who eat them in large enough quantities. So if you decide that you want your protein intake to consist of meat, poultry, eggs, or dairy, make sure that you are purchasing organic items. They are free of toxic chemicals and hormones. You can obtain organic dairy products and eggs at many supermarkets, and at most health food stores. Make sure these products are labeled "Certified Organic." This new, government-required label assures you that the item you are purchasing is indeed authentically organic since, in the past, the word *organic* was used loosely and freely, without quality control or consumer protection.

Make sure, also, that your animal products are lean. Trim the fat off your meat and skin your chicken. Grill, don't fry. Drink organic skim milk and cook primarily with organic egg whites instead of whole eggs if you need to lower your cholesterol intake.

Fish is an underused but extremely important form of protein. As mentioned above, fish oil has its own set of benefits. Fish may be a superior form of protein because it does not contain antibiotics or growth hormones, and is considerably lower in fat than other forms of animal protein. If possible try to obtain farm-raised fish, because it comes from water free of pollutants and toxins.

You may be surprised to learn that you can "overdo" your consumption of even the healthiest forms of protein. An excessive intake of protein can contribute to bone loss by causing calcium to be excreted in the urine. You can counteract this insidious effect by eating larger quantities of protein-rich soy foods that actually boost bone health. As a peri- and postmenopausal woman, these will be the most important sources of protein for you, because of their high phytoestrogen and easy-to-absorb calcium content.

You should eat between three and five servings of protein per day. Each serving should consist of approximately three to six ounces, or 85 to 170 grams. Table 3:2 lists some of the most common sources of protein, and what constitutes a serving of each.

Table 3:2 Protein Servings

Food	Quantity/Measurement
Egg (whole)	1
Egg (whites)	1
Chicken breast	3–4 oz
Chicken drumstick	3–4 oz
Turkey breast	3–4 oz
Turkey drumstick	3–4 oz
Tofu	6 oz
Veggie burger	5 oz
Fish (grilled)	4 oz
Fish (canned)	4–6 oz
Seafood	4–6 medium shrimp
Sardines	4–6 oz
Lean veal	4–6 oz
Soy milk	1 cup
Rice milk	1 cup
Skim milk	1 cup
Yogurt	6–8 oz
Cottage cheese	4–6 oz
Beans (soy, garbanzo)	1/2 cup

Note: If you wish, you can substitute red meat, pork, or lamb for 1 protein serving with 1–2 meals/week.

Carbohydrates

Carbohydrates are foods that provide your body with energy. They can be classified into two basic categories: simple and complex.

Sugars and highly refined starches like white-flour products consist exclusively of simple carbohydrates. Beans, whole grains, and vegetables, on the other hand, contain complex carbohydrates. Fruits contain both simple and complex carbohydrates, although the complex form predominates.

Both simple and complex carbohydrates are eventually broken down by the body into their basic component—glucose. This is the form of sugar that is converted into usable energy by the insulin that your pancreas produces. When the energy is not used immediately, it is stored in your body's cells as fat. (Now you know why you gain weight when you eat too much cake or chocolate.)

Even though all carbohydrates—simple and complex—are ultimately broken down into glucose, there are significant differences in how the various forms of carbohydrates are metabolized. Simple carbohydrates are absorbed immediately by the body. They arrive in a ready-made form and are instantaneously converted by the body into energy. You experience a "rush" and a "high." But then you suddenly feel an energy drop, or a "crash," when the impact of the sugar has worn off. Your pancreas has poured large quantities of insulin into the bloodstream to handle the enormous onslaught of sugar. The insulin, having done its job, remains in the bloodstream and can lead to irritability. The body has also expended a great deal of energy and feels understandably drained and exhausted.

Complex carbohydrates, on the other hand, work like time-released energy pills. Fuel is sustained and energy levels rise slowly, as the body works hard and takes time breaking down the carbohydrates and releasing the energy gradually. Moreover, a large proportion of the simple carbohydrates you eat are immediately converted into fat by the body and stored in your fat cells. The metabolic process of conversion and storage is considerably slower in the case of complex carbohydrates. This allows your body to process and dispose of excess before it can be stowed away in unsightly cells lining your thighs, hips, and buttocks.

Complex carbohydrates—such as whole grains, fruits, and vegetables—have a few additional benefits. They are rich in vitamins, minerals, fiber, and all sorts of phytonutrients that play a crucial role in building good health and preventing illness. We will discuss these further as we look at each carbohydrate source and what it can contribute to your peri- and postmenopausal health.

I have had overweight patients react with alarm when I have told them that they must eat a certain amount of carbohydrates—whole grains, legumes, and starchy vegetables—in order to stay healthy and lose weight. "But bread, potatoes, and rice are fattening!" they protest.

I explain to these patients that scientists have recently discovered that reasonable quantities of these carbohydrates aren't fattening and are far better for your body than too much fat or even too much protein. I add that refined carbohydrates—white toast, pasta, processed mashed potatoes, or white rice, for example—*are* fattening, and are almost as detrimental to your health as refined sugar. They don't contain enough fiber, and most of their vitamins and minerals have been leached out through the refinement process. The kind of carbohydrate that will not add weight is complex rather than refined. When it comes to bread, and rice, the only kind that will contribute to a shapely figure and good health is the whole-grain, high-fiber product.

Whole, unprocessed grains are healthy and satisfying complex carbohydrates. They are rich in nutrients such as B vitamins, magnesium, zinc, iron, calcium, and protein. Whole grains also contain plenty of fiber. Brown rice, whole oats, rye, barley, wheat, bulgur wheat, and corn are excellent grains. They are versatile, filling, and nutritious.

Please note that some of the so-called whole-wheat bread you might buy at the supermarket doesn't qualify as an unprocessed grain product. It's almost as refined as cotton-wool white bread. My whole-grain bread—which I purchase at the health food store—feels almost as heavy as the weights I lift when I work out.

You may be wondering how to tell the difference between authentic "whole-grain products" and those that claim to be whole grain, but are not superior to refined products. Do you have to bring a scale or lift them in your hands?

Not at all. The package of bread or cereal should give you all the information you need. When you are reading the label, investigate how much total dietary fiber is contained in the product you're buying. Your whole-grain bread should contain at least four grams of fiber per slice. (That rules out most commercial breads and sends you to the health food store rather than the supermarket for your sandwich needs.) Cereal should contain at least five grams of fiber per serving. Table 3:3 will show you what constitutes a "serving" of many different types of complex carbohydrates.

It is especially important to read labels now that the FDA has authorized cereal companies and others to use the term *whole grain* on the packages of many popular items that have virtually no fiber at all! As in so many other areas of your health, you must be an educated consumer and read not only the boldly stated claims but also the fine print on the products you buy.

Whole grains are an important source of carbohydrates but are by no means the only one. While there are cultures (particularly in Asia) where rice, for example, constitutes virtually the sole source of carbohydrates, we live in a society where more variety is available. This variety enhances our health because starchy vegetables and legumes contain phytonutrients not present in grains. So when you decide what to eat each day, try to vary your menu. You might have a whole-grain cereal for breakfast and a whole-wheat sandwich for lunch—but then you should try to choose your evening starch from among the starchy vegetables and legume category. Unskinned potatoes, yams, beets, winter squash, and beans are examples of starchy vegetables. They are excellent sources of complex carbohydrates, as well as other phytohormones and phytonutrients that are anticarcinogenic and that help fight cardiovascular disease. So are legumes such as peas and beans.

Garbanzo beans—also called chickpeas—deserve special mention here because they are such a rich source of phytoestrogens, as we discussed above. Garbanzo beans are quite versatile. Mediterranean cultures use them extensively in such dishes as falafel. Humus is an excellent way to serve chickpeas, because it combines them with tahini—a paste made out of sesame butter. Sesame seeds are high in protein.

Soy also deserves special mention—yet again. It is unique because it is the only complete source of vegetable protein. It is also rich in fiber and other phytonutrients. Best of all—from a culinary point of view—it's extremely versatile. You can do all sorts of amazing things with soy, adding flavor, variety, and nutrition to all your meals.

You should try to eat three to five servings of complex carbohydrates daily. You should avoid refined carbohydrates as much as possible.

Table 3:3 will show you how much of each complex carbohydrate constitutes a serving.

Table 3:3 Complex Carbohydrate Servings

Legumes and Starchy Vegetables	
Baked beans	1/2 cup
Beans (cooked)	1/2 cup
Beets	1/2 cup
Garbanzo beans	1/2 cup
Corn	1/2 cup
Corn on the cob	1 ear
Lima beans	1/2 cup
Parsnips	1/2 cup
Peas, green	1/2 cup
Lentils	1/2 cup
Plantain	1/2 cup
Potato, baked	1/2 large
Potato, mashed	1/2 cup
Pumpkin	1/2 cup
Soybeans	1/2 cup
Squash, winter	1/2 cup
Squash, spaghetti	1/2 cup
Sweet potato	1/2 large
Yam	1/2 large
Cooked Grains	
Rice (whole-grain/wild)	1/3 cup
Pasta (whole-grain)	1/2 cup
Popcorn (air-popped)	3 cups
Bulgur wheat	1/2 cup
Couscous (whole-grain)	1/2 cup
Kasha	1/2 cup
Bread/Crackers (Choose whole-grain, high-fiber products)	
Whole-wheat	1 slice
Rye	1 slice

Pumpernickel	1 slice
Raisin	1 slice
Multigrain	1 slice
Bagel	1/2
English muffin	1/2
Roll	1 small
Pita bread	1 small
Hot dog/hamburger bun	1/2
Bread crumbs	1/2 cup
Tortilla	1 small
Croutons (toasted)	1 cup
Pancake	1
Waffle	1
High-fiber crackers	3–5
Cereal	
All Bran	1/2 cup
Bran Flakes	1/2 cup
Shredded wheat	1/2 cup
Oatmeal	1/2 cup
Cream of Wheat	1/2 cup
Cream of rice	1/2 cup
Wheat germ	1 tbsp.
Muesli (sugar-free)	1/2 cup

Fruits   Fruits are sweet, delicious, and highly nutritious carbohydrates. While they are metabolized far more quickly than grains and for that reason should be eaten in moderation, they are also high in phytoestrogens, vitamins, and many other nutrients. All fresh fruits contain useful vitamins, such as vitamin A, vitamin B6, and vitamin C; and essential minerals such as potassium and boron; and other important nutrients. Try to consume two to three servings of whole fruit each day. Table 3:4 will tell you what constitutes a "serving" of fruit. Juice should be diluted with water or seltzer and used sparingly.

Table 3:4 Fruit Servings

Apple	1 medium
Apples, dried	4 rings
Applesauce (fresh)	1/2 cup
Apricots	4 medium
Banana	1/2, or 1 small
Blackberries	3/4 cup
Boysenberries	3/4 cup
Cantaloupe	1/3
Cherries	12 large
Figs, fresh	2
Fresh fruit cup	1/2 cup
Grapes	15
Grapefruit	1/2
Grapefruit juice (fresh)	1/2 cup
Guava	1 small
Honeydew	1/6 medium
Kiwi	1 large
Lemon	1 large
Mango	1/2 small
Nectarine	1 medium
Orange	1 medium
Orange juice (fresh)	1/2 cup
Passion fruit	3/4 cup
Peach	1 medium
Pear	1 small
Pineapple	1/2 cup
Pineapple juice (fresh)	1/2 cup
Plums	2
Pomegranate	1/2
Raspberries	3/4 cup
Strawberries	3/4 cup

It is important to eat cut or squeezed fruits when they are actually fresh, not when they have sat around all day. The fruit salad you get at a restaurant, salad bar, or supermarket has lost most of its nutrients, since it's prepared en masse in the morning. "Freshly squeezed orange juice" may be called "fresh" because it doesn't come from a carton or can, but that doesn't mean it's actually fresh. Make sure it has been squeezed within the hour, or you'll lose most of the vitamin C.

When you eat a whole piece of fruit, you are also consuming fiber. Fiber is what slows the absorption of the natural sugars contained in fruit. Some people may find that fruit juice—even if it is unsweetened—overloads the system with simple carbohydrates because it is usually devoid of any fiber. (This includes the "pulpy" variety of orange juice in cartons lining the dairy case.) Too many fruit juices can be almost as detrimental as too much candy.

Finally, vary your fruit intake so that you can get a wide variety of vitamins, minerals, and other phytonutrients. An apple a day probably won't keep the doctor away; but an apple on Monday, a peach on Tuesday, and a banana on Wednesday may do the trick. I always advise my patients to eat a rainbow of fruits and vegetables—orange, green, yellow, red, and blue. Remembering to vary your colors will help you to eat a broad range of different phytonutrients.

Vegetables   If there is a single food group associated with good health, it's probably vegetables. (Mom was right again.) Scarcely a day goes by when some venerable scientific institution hasn't published a study associating high vegetable consumption with some area of health, and with diminished risk of disease. Some of these studies are cited in the References section for this chapter (page 186).

I have divided vegetables into two categories—nonstarchy and starchy. While both grow in the ground and are therefore called "vegetables," and both are available in the same aisle of the supermarket, starchy vegetables are metabolized quite differently from nonstarchy ones. A potato, yam, or butternut squash is metabolized like a cup of rice or a slice of whole-grain bread rather than like a stalk of broccoli or a leaf of lettuce. When you are planning out your day's meals, you will want to have at least six servings of nonstarchy vegetables each day. The guiding principle when it comes to nonstarchy vegetables is this: the more, the merrier. The suggestions in this book are minimum rather than maximum quantities. The more broccoli, collard greens, carrots, and cabbage you eat, the healthier you'll be. That's not the case with potatoes or yams, which can add undesirable weight if eaten in excess. Starchy vegetables must be budgeted in the same category with grains and legumes.

Nonstarchy vegetables include carrots, celery, collard greens, lettuce, summer squash, tomatoes, and a host of other nutritious produce. You should have at least six servings of these vegetables each day. A serving consists of a cup of cooked vegetables, or a cup of salad.

The Importance of Fiber   Fiber isn't just for genteel elderly people who appear in television commercials talking in euphemistic terms about becoming more "regular." Fiber is essential for everybody. It serves several important purposes. To begin with, fiber slows the absorption of naturally occurring sugar in foods, so that you don't experience the "rush" and "crash" effect we discussed earlier. The digestive system must work hard to dispose of the unusable materials in order to absorb the usable materials and, in so doing, the process takes longer. This prevents the "rush" effect that sugar and refined grain products create, with its accompanying mood swings and stress upon the pancreas.

Fiber also "scrubs" the inside of the intestines, making sure that debris does not accumulate along the intestinal walls. This goes a long way toward reducing the risk of colon cancer and other gastrointestinal disorders such as diverticulosis (the formation of pockets in the bowel) and diverticulitis (an infection that occurs when food becomes trapped in these pockets, allowing bacteria to grow).

Finally, fiber adds bulk to the stool. This renders bowel movements more regular and also easier to pass, thereby reducing the risk of hemorrhoids and anal fissures. A high-fiber diet can trap cholesterol and fat, thereby reducing these levels in blood. Also, a high-fiber diet can help reduce high estradiol levels by trapping and excreting excess estradiol in the stool.

You should be eating 25 grams of fiber every day. You can accomplish this by increasing your consumption of unprocessed grain products, whole fruits and vegetables, and bran. You will find out exactly how much fiber is present in the packaged foods you eat by studying the labels. Look at the panel of food ingredients and nutrients, and see how much total dietary fiber is present in the item you're about to purchase or eat. Try to vary the types of fiber foods you eat to include a mix of soluble and insoluble fiber.

If you want to augment your intake of fiber, you can add oat bran or wheat germ to dishes such as yogurt, cold cereal, hot cereal, casseroles, and meat loaf (preferably made from ground lean beef or turkey). This is an easy way to slip additional fiber into the diet of the entire family.

The Importance of Water

Water is an essential part of your daily diet. Most professionals agree that you should try to consume close to eight cups of water each day. You do not, however, need to gulp down eight full glasses of water. It is possible for you to get some of your water intake (usually up to three glasses) from the water present in fruits and vegetables. Juice, tea, and soup also contain substantial quantities of water.

Make sure the water you drink is spring, mineral, or filtered water rather than water straight from the tap. Most of our municipal water is contaminated with chemicals and even parasites from time to time, and should be avoided. Even boiling does not remove all of the toxins. You can obtain water filters that attach to your faucet, or you can buy smaller and less expensive pitcher units that will filter your water right in your refrigerator.

Your New Diet at a Glance

This chapter contains a great deal of new material. I know that it's a lot to take in all at once. To make things easier for you, here is an at-a-glance summary of the dietary recommendations I've discussed in this chapter. I hope that these tips will help you to organize and remember what you've learned.

Balance Your Omega-3 and Omega-6 Fatty Acids

Reduce your intake of saturated and hydrogenated fats, such as those present in red meats, butter, hard cheese, and commercial cookies and crackers. Limit your intake of omega-6 fatty acids by minimizing your use of vegetable oils, shortenings, margarine, and mayonnaise. When you must cook with oil, use unprocessed canola, olive, or safflower oil in your cooking—and only in limited quantities. Make sure you get two tablespoons of an omega-3 fatty acid several times a week. You can do this by eating a diet rich in vegetables, fruits, whole grains, and fatty fish such as salmon. Nuts and seeds—especially flaxseed—will also supply you with this type of healthy oil.

Include Three to Five Servings of Protein Every Day

You should eat between three and five servings of protein per day. Each serving should consist of approximately three to six ounces, or 85 to 170 grams. When you are selecting your protein, be sure it comes in the most healthful form possible. So choose farm-raised fish whenever it is available, and make sure your meat, poultry, and dairy products are certified organic. Your meat should be lean, your poultry should be skin-free, and your milk should be skim or low-fat. Soy products provide the most superior form of protein because they are high in phytoestrogens and low in fat. As with other foods, if you can obtain organic soy products, you are ensuring a higher-quality, lower-toxin item.

Include Three to Five Servings of Complex Starchy Carbohydrates Every Day

Vary your starch intake to include whole grains, starchy vegetables, and legumes. These provide a varied array of phytonutrients, as well as a diverse menu so that you don't get bored with any single food item. It is advisable to include at least one serving of soybeans or garbanzo beans daily, because they are high in protein and phytoestrogens.

Include At Least Six Servings of Nonstarchy Vegetables Every Day

Your vegetable intake should include both cooked and raw vegetables. If you eat a large salad every day, you will be taking in a variety of wonderful phytonutrients in their freshest form. Cooked vegetables, such as broccoli, collard greens, kale, and cauliflower, will provide you with different but equally important nutrients.

Here are a few important caveats to keep in mind:

- *Remember the rainbow.* If you eat a rainbow of colors each day—orange carrots, red tomatoes, yellow squash, purple eggplant, green broccoli—you will be sure to take in a wide range of rich phytonutrients.
- *Never overcook your vegetables.* You will leach the nutrients out of your vegetables if you overcook them. They should be lightly steamed, rather than boiled. Three to four minutes' cooking time is usually suf-

ficient. Remember that they should be on the crisp side, rather than soft and mushy.

- *Make sure fresh vegetables are really fresh.* Many of the salads you buy at "salad bars" have sat out since the wee hours, when a bleary-eyed chef prepared them for the day's customers. Fresh vegetables should be crisp and bright colored. Avoid wilted, sad-looking vegetables, and if you have any questions, ask the waiter how long ago the vegetables were cut or diced. If they've been standing around for more than two hours, they've probably lost most of their nutritional content.

Drink Eight Cups of Filtered or Bottled Water or the Equivalent Every Day

Keep yourself well hydrated, even in cool weather and especially in the summer heat. Carrying a water bottle with you often helps to remind you to drink. Juices and herbal teas can be substituted for water. Remember, however, that too much juice—even unsweetened—can raise blood sugar levels and can also be fattening.

Eat Two to Three Servings of Fruit Each Day

Fruits are as important as vegetables, but should be eaten in smaller quantities. Although they are high in phytonutrients, their high sugar content means they have to be eaten sparingly. Here are a few caveats to remember:

- *Raw is better than cooked.* A cooked fruit loses most of its nutrients. From a metabolic point of view, cooked fruit—especially if consumed in excessive quantities—acts more like a simple than a complex carbohydrate. It is metabolized rapidly, often contributing to the "rise-then-crash" phenomenon, and is also more likely to contribute to weight gain.
- *Whole fruit is better than juice.* Fruit juices are often devoid of important nutrients. Moreover, the removal of most of the fiber means that they are metabolized like simple rather than complex carbohydrates.
- *Buy organic fruit.* Fruits are usually treated with pesticides. Many have been subjected to additional chemicals to "fast-ripen" them. Still other fruits are imported from countries that do not observe standards of

pesticide safety comparable to those demanded by the FDA. So as often as possible, purchase certified organic produce. When that is not possible, try to buy fruits at a local farmer's market, where you can inquire from the growers what chemicals were used in the agricultural process. Try to buy fruits in season. Out-of-season produce has probably been imported from other countries. And always be sure to wash your produce thoroughly under running water, so as to remove as much pesticide residue as possible.

Modifying Your Diet . . . One Step at a Time

Food is central to our culture. We have only to walk through the streets of any major city and count the restaurants to see what an important role food plays in our society. We conduct business meetings at lunch and treat ourselves to an evening off by going out to dinner. Families meet to bond or argue at mealtime, and the lives of many women revolve around the kitchen and the table. Women approaching midlife have evolved culinary and dietary habits and practices that reflect their lifestyles. Asking women to alter long-standing practices—often of twenty or thirty years' duration—can elicit distressed, almost panicky responses.

Indeed, some of my patients react with dismay when I tell them that they have to make changes to their diet. They groan, anticipating a complicated and overwhelming new series of chores as they learn to do without their fast-food breakfasts and their TV dinners. Many also resent having to give up their favorite foods (or cooking differently, so that their husbands and children give up their favorite foods). Some even worry that they will never enjoy eating again!

I can only assure them—and you—that this isn't the case. Altering your dietary habits isn't a complicated task at all, and eating doesn't have to become a dull experience. There are some excellent books available that can help you create easy-to-prepare, delicious, and nutritious meals. Some of these books are listed in Resources (page 195).

Below you will find some suggestions to help you get a handle on the process of dietary modification. There's no need to turn the kitchen upside down. Start with some simple changes and put them into effect one at a time. After a few weeks or months of becoming accustomed to the modification, move to the next one. Here are a few suggestions:

- Substitute fish for meat a few times a week.
- Incorporate a soy product into your diet a few times a week.
- Add vegetables—cooked as well as raw—to your diet. Perhaps this will involve carrying carrot sticks to work and munching them on the bus. Perhaps you will start to have a salad for lunch, or an additional serving of broccoli for dinner. Vegetable soup with rice makes a delicious hot breakfast that will provide you with a steadier and more reliable energy boost than cereal and milk, or coffee and danish.
- When the craving for something sweet strikes, nibble on a piece of fruit, such as an apple or a banana. Fruit tastes wonderful and will satisfy your "sugar munchies."
- Substitute low-fat for high-fat products. For example, let's say you and your family have enjoyed ice cream for dessert a few times a week. You can substitute low-fat frozen yogurt. You can obtain many delicious organic brands and flavors at the health food store. You can also substitute all-fruit (no sugar added) organic sorbet—likewise available at the health food store.
- Find stores in your area that carry certified organic products, and do your shopping at these stores. More and more supermarkets are now stocking organic dairy products—especially milk—as well as organic produce. No longer does "organic" connote a few shriveled gray oranges in a bin at the health food store. Organic fruits and vegetables are as colorful and succulent as their chemical-laden counterparts. Often, they taste better because they have not been fast-gassed for rapid ripening, nor have they been subjected to chemicals that can seep into the produce and alter its flavor. Organic cereals, cookies, and other products are also becoming available in supermarkets, and an even wider variety is available at health food stores.

These suggestions, taken one at a time, will help you to move gently but steadily toward healthier eating. If you undertake each step in its good time, you have increased your chances that your new, health-embracing modification will remain with you beyond menopause and well into your senior years.

Diet: Your Key to Menopausal Health

We have seen that a well-balanced diet supplies your body with many necessary nutrients. These nutrients—especially phytoestrogens—assist your body in stabilizing hormonal levels, and thereby reduce uncomfortable symptoms such as hot flashes and vaginal dryness. They build healthy bones and heart, and render HRT something superfluous at best, and completely unnecessary.

Correct eating is necessary and powerful, but is not the only factor in your overall menopause program. Chapter 4 will discuss nutritional supplements and other dietary means of enhancing your health. If you take them together with normal, manageable quantities of soy and vegetables, you will be well on your way to a total program of menopausal well-being.

Foods to Limit or Eliminate

By now you've probably figured out much of the following section, but it's worth reviewing. So many of the products I'm about to list constitute staples of the average American diet that it's particularly important to understand how detrimental they are, and why I'm asking you to give up some of your favorite foods.

Of course, you can indulge in them every now and then. It's fun and healthy to be able to enjoy yourself when you're at a party, or when you're having dinner with friends. Most of the time, the problem doesn't lie in the occasional fling, but rather in the daily assault on the system that takes place when people regularly consume unhealthy foods. If your daily diet consists of a caffeine-and-danish breakfast, a mayonnaise-and-white-bread lunch, and a pasta-and-steak dinner, you will suffer ill effects sooner or later, both because you are not eating healthy foods like vegetables and fiber, and because you are flooding your system with sugars, fats, and chemical toxins.

Dairy Products

Many of us grew up being taught that "milk builds strong bones." This may be true of breast milk, but it's not true of cow's milk. We're not cows, and large quantities of cow's milk do not agree with most of us. Part of the problem is that cows are fed bovine growth hormone to aid in their milk production and growth. This hormone upsets the human hormonal balance, so important to maintain during the menopausal years. Moreover, our bodies often rebel against the lactose (milk sugar) in milk. Lactose-intolerant individuals suffer from a variety of digestive disturbances if they've drunk milk. There is also strong anecdotal evidence pointing to the role that milk may play in increasing mucus secretions, especially in individuals who suffer from asthma or allergies. My own clinical experience certainly confirms this connection, and I always advise clients with respiratory difficulties—such as colds, coughs, bronchitis, and sinusitis—to avoid dairy products.

Most postmenopausal American women are encouraged to consume large quantities of dairy so as to increase their calcium intake, because calcium loss is responsible for osteoporosis. They have been convinced that dairy is the only source of dietary calcium, and that the more dairy they eat, the healthier their bones will be.

It's certainly true that dairy products contain calcium. But dairy is by no means the only, or even the superior, source of calcium. In fact, the calcium contained in dairy is not presented to your body in the most useful form. Like many other minerals, calcium is best absorbed by the body when taken in combination with several other minerals. These include vitamin D, magnesium, zinc, copper, boron, and manganese—none of which is present in milk, cheese, or yogurt. There are also phytonutrients that aid in the absorption and usability of calcium. These include two isoflavones called genistein and daidzein.

Here's another interesting fact: studies have shown that Japanese women, who eat a native diet rich in soy, have the lowest incidence of hip fracture. While they do get some calcium in their diet from soy and other sources, they certainly do not drink large quantities of milk. Apparently, their bones are strengthened by noncalcium nutrients, such as boron, manganese, copper, magnesium, genistein, and daidzein. All these can greatly increase bone density. Table 3:5 suggests some excellent non-

dairy sources of calcium and other bone-building nutrients and phytonutrients, and tells you how much of each constitutes a serving. I recommend that you eat two to three servings of bone-building compounds
daily.

Table 3:5 Nondairy Sources of Calcium

Food	Serving Size
Tofu	1/2 cup
Soy milk	6–8 oz
Soybeans (cooked)	1 cup
Salmon	4–6 oz
Mackerel	4–6 oz
Sardines	4–6 oz
Shrimp	4–6 medium
Kale	1 cup
Collard greens	1 cup
Spinach	1 cup
Broccoli	1 cup
Black beans	1 cup
Winter squash	1 cup
White beans	1 cup

Sugar and Refined Grain Products

It's interesting to note that in nature, sweeteners are hard to come by and
require some effort to collect and process. If you wish to suck sugarcane
juice, you must fight your way through dense fields and cut away all sorts
of greenery before finally accessing the sweet interior of the canes. You
must climb a tree to pick its fruit, drill a hole to extract its syrup, or battle the bees to obtain honey. In the premodern world, sugars were therefore a great luxury and were consumed sparingly. Maybe Nature was
trying to tell us something by making sugar so inaccessible. The message
is probably this: Don't eat too much sugar!

Aside from causing all sorts of dental problems, sugar wreaks havoc with the body's metabolism. It elevates blood sugar levels rapidly. Then, when the effects have worn off, there is a "crash" as the blood sugar levels plunge. The fluctuations in blood sugar levels, in turn, overtax the pancreas. And of course, too much sugar—whether in the form of candy, soda, cake, white bread, or white pasta—adds extra weight. In fact, obesity has become an American epidemic! Indulge once in a while, but avoid regular and frequent consumption of sugar and white-flour products.

High-Fat Products

As mentioned earlier, red meat, fatty poultry, ice cream, whole milk, excessive quantities of egg yolks, fried foods, fast food, and junk food are high in fat, which adds undesirable weight. This weight is unsightly and also quite detrimental to your general and postmenopausal health. Too much fat can increase the number and size of fat cells, thereby elevating estradiol levels in the body. Finally, it increases the risk of cardiovascular disease and many forms of cancer. I have heard many patients protest that their partners are "meat and potatoes" men who must have their steak and fries. These women complain that they don't want to cook "just for themselves." I urge my patients to begin loving themselves by eating healthful foods, no matter how their partners feel about it. I also tell them that they're not doing their partners a favor by serving foods that endanger cardiovascular health.

Foods with Chemicals, Pesticides, or Additives

Here's a good dictum to follow: The more natural a product, the more healthy it is likely to be. Chemical preservatives, pesticides, or other additives contain many toxic substances such as heavy metals that are known to be carcinogenic. Studies have linked these toxins with cancer, respiratory problems, and neurological disorders in children as well as adults. As much as possible, try to avoid them.

Food Versus Supplements

If you are like some of my patients, you may be wondering why you need to eat healthful foods if you can find such a wide variety of excellent nutritional supplements available in your health food store.

You can certainly supply your body with some major nutrients by taking supplements. Indeed, we will be looking at many of these supplements in chapter 4. But there are important phytonutrients that must be supplied through diet. Science is at the beginning of the long process of isolating particular plant compounds that are responsible for particular effects in the body. Scientists are starting to understand which phytonutrients protect against cancer, for example, or against heart disease. But people have been eating for thousands of years, and the wide range of rich phytonutrients available in whole, unprocessed foods belies even the most skillful scientific research and nutritional supplementation. If you were to supplement every one of the presently known phytonutrients in amounts that would be useful to your body, you'd be consuming vast quantities of pills and powders, and would not even begin to approximate what's available in a well-balanced diet. What you can purchase in a health food store constitutes a tiny fraction of the thousands of varied phytonutrients contained in a single bite of good food.

Here's another reason to get your nutritional needs from food as much as possible: Food tastes better than pills!

On the other hand, supplementation is important. The agricultural conditions responsible for the growth of our produce and our other foods and the processing procedures to which our food is subjected often drain some of the nutrients from the food. Food may contain nutrients you cannot find in supplements, but supplements supply nutrients often not found in food. The optimum daily requirements of important vitamins, minerals, and other nutrients are not always present in the foods we eat. The most effective approach to health involves integrating a complete, well-balanced diet with a complete, well-balanced program of supplementation.

Four

Nutritional Supplements to Help
You Avoid the Roller Coaster

For all too many of us, diet and exercise are not sufficient to address perimenopausal symptoms such as hot flashes, fatigue, or vaginal dryness.
Postmenopausal conditions such as cardiovascular disease and osteoporosis are even more serious, and often require treatment that goes beyond what unassisted diet and exercise can accomplish.

This chapter will introduce you to powerful and effective supplements
that can help you prevent or reverse perimenopausal discomforts and
postmenopausal disorders. You will learn which vitamins, minerals, nutritional supplements, and herbs will be most useful in addressing your
complaints. You will learn the name of each item, what symptoms it addresses, and how to use it. The charts at the end of the chapter (page
122) will help you organize this information into a systematic guide
to handling your particular constellation of perimenopausal and postmenopausal symptoms.

Vitamins and Minerals

Vitamins and minerals are nutrients that are essential to life. They are often called micronutrients because, in comparison with the other major
food groups, they are utilized by the body only in relatively small quantities.

While vitamins and minerals are present in many of the foods you eat,
it is virtually impossible to meet all your nutritional needs by eating the

food available to us today. People who try to eat a "well-balanced diet" often are misinformed regarding the actual nutritional content of the foods they eat—much of which is overstated or exaggerated by claims on the package label. Moreover, the nutritional content of foods—especially where minerals are concerned—fluctuates widely, depending on the growing conditions of the food item. Our soil is depleted of many minerals, and some of the most commonly used fertilizers do not supply adequate quantities of nutritionally rich plant food. The length of time it takes for a fruit or vegetable to reach us, the method of storage, and the processing techniques further deplete the food item of its nutrients. There are few people in the United States today who do not require vitamin and mineral supplementation.

Perimenopausal and postmenopausal women have additional needs. Let's look at the vitamins and minerals that are important in addressing some of the most common conditions.

Multivitamin-Multimineral Supplements

All women should take a good-quality general multivitamin product that supplies substantial quantities of basic vitamins and minerals. These are easily available in health food stores, and in many supermarkets and pharmacies. There is an overwhelming number of products from which you can choose, and it's easy to become confused or overwhelmed by the vast selection. All products are not alike, however. Here are a few pointers and tips for selecting the best-quality product:

Natural Versus Synthetic   Make sure your multivitamin supplement comes from natural sources. While the superiority of natural over synthetic remains controversial in terms of nutritional content, one thing is clear: A product labeled "natural" does not contain unnatural ingredients such as coal tar, artificial coloring, preservatives, sugar, starch, or other additives. These ingredients are unnecessary, and might even be detrimental.

Vitamin and Mineral Contents   A basic multivitamin and multimineral supplement should contain minimum dosages of the most important vitamins and minerals. Table 4:1 will give you some general idea of what to look for. You may not find a single multivitamin-multimineral supplement that conforms to an exact set of suggested levels, so any product with levels falling within the ranges listed below is acceptable. Some vitamins, such as vitamin A, are measured in terms of international units (IUs). Others are measured in milligrams (mgs). Still others are measured in micrograms (mcgs). Beta-carotene may be measured as mgs or IUs. For simplicity's sake, this book uses international units.

Table 4:1 What to Look For in a Multivitamin-Multimineral Supplement

Vitamin/Mineral	Amount per Tablet
Vitamin A	5,000–10,000 IU
Beta-carotene	10,000–25,000 IU
Vitamin C	500–1,000 mg
Vitamin D	400–800 IU
Vitamin E	200–600 IU
Thiamin	50–100 mg
Riboflavin	50–100 mg
Niacin	50–100 mg
Vitamin B6	50–100 mg
Folic Acid	400–800 mcg
Vitamin B12	50–100 mcg
Biotin	10–50 mcg
Pantothenic Acid	10–50 mg
Inositol	10–25 mg
PABA	10–25 mg
Calcium	500–1,000 mg
Magnesium	250–500 mg
Zinc	15–50 mg
Copper	0.5–2 mg
Manganese	5–15 mg
Boron	1–3 mg
Selenium	50–200 mcg
Iodine	50–150 mcg
Chromium	50–200 mcg

A Note About Storage   Supplements do not last forever. Their potency gradually diminishes over time. Always buy supplements with an expiration date stamped clearly on the label, and use the product before that date.

Supplements should be stored in a cool, dark place. The refrigerator is too cold and too moist for maximum potency to be sustained, so I don't recommend it as a storage place. Many people like to keep their supplements on top of the refrigerator—this is also a problem. The refrigerator motor generates heat and is too warm for effective vitamin storage. A room-temperature closet is usually fine.

If you wish to transfer your supplements to a small container for work or travel, make sure it is opaque and closes tightly. You can store your supplements for several months without worrying about loss of potency.

Vitamin Supplements for Menopause

Over and above the vitamins you need to keep you in generally good health, there are specific vitamins that will help you to address certain conditions and discomforts. You might want to increase your intake of these vitamins during the perimenopausal and postmenopausal years, according to the nature and severity of your symptoms. Here are the most important vitamins.

Vitamin A and Beta-Carotene

Vitamin A performs many important functions in your body. It builds resistance to illness and protects you from cardiovascular disease and cancer. It also plays an important role in maintaining the good health of your skin and eyes.

The components that form vitamin A fall into two groups—the *retinoids* (preformed vitamin A) and the *carotenoids* (precursors of vitamin A that your body converts into active and usable vitamin A). Beta-carotene is the most important—and also the most scientifically studied—carotenoid.

Vitamin A and beta-carotene are particularly useful for women during the years before and after menopause, because they strengthen mucous membranes. If you are suffering from vaginal dryness or atrophy, vitamin A and beta-carotene will help strengthen the interior of your vaginal wall.

Supplements I generally recommend that my patients take a combination of natural beta-carotene and active vitamin A. While you can usually get enough vitamin A in your multivitamin supplement, if you are experiencing the symptoms discussed above and you need to supplement, I advise you to find a mixed carotenoid supplement. This includes beta-carotene and other naturally occurring carotenoids, which are precursors to vitamin A in your system.

Recommended Dosage For optimum general health, the basic Optimum Daily Intake for vitamin A is 5,000–10,000 IU (the amount usually found in a good multivitamin). For beta-carotene, it is 11,000–50,000 IU (most will be found in your multivitamin).

Based on a thorough scientific review of vitamin A and beta-carotene, and on my clinical experience, the following amounts of vitamin A and beta-carotene appear to be valuable for:

Condition	Suggested Dosage Vitamin A	Suggested Dosage Beta-Carotene
Vaginal dryness	10,000–25,000 IU	25,000–50,000 IU

Toxicity and Adverse Effects All forms of vitamin A—both fat- and water-soluble—are stored in the liver. Vitamin A can therefore be toxic in large amounts. In general, a healthy adult must take at least 100,000 IU of vitamin A daily for a period of months in order to display any signs of toxicity. Early warning signs are fatigue, nausea, headache, vertigo, blurred vision, lack of muscular coordination, and loss of body hair.

Beta-carotene, on the other hand, can be taken for long periods without any risk of toxicity. Since beta-carotene is a naturally occurring pigment, the only adverse effect of taking too much is the possibility of carotenemia—a harmless condition in which the skin turns a slight orange color, signaling that the body has converted as much beta-carotene as it can.

The B Vitamins

The vitamins that belong to the B-complex group are B_1 (thiamin), B_2 (riboflavin), B_3 (niacin and niacinamide), B_6 (pyridoxine), B_{12} (cobalamin), folic acid, pantothenic acid, biotin, choline, inositol, and PABA (para-aminobenzoic acid). Each B vitamin has its own unique biological role to play and its own individual properties. They all have so much in common, however, that they are generally thought of as being a single entity.

For menopausal women, the most important function of the B vitamin group is the alleviation of emotional symptoms, such as anxiety and depression. Specific B vitamins are also useful in lowering the levels of blood cholesterol and triglycerides, reducing symptoms of bloating and breast tenderness associated with hormonal fluctuations, and addressing arthritis and anemia.

Supplements   I usually recommend a complete vitamin B-complex supplement.

Recommended Dosage   For optimum general health, the basic Optimum Daily Intake for vitamin B is:

Vitamin B_1	50–100 mg
Vitamin B_2	50–100 mg
Vitamin B_3	50–100 mg
Vitamin B_6	50–100 mg
Vitamin B_{12}	50–100 mcg
Folic Acid	400–800 mcg

Based on a thorough scientific review of vitamin B complex, and on my clinical experience, the following amounts of vitamin B complex appear to be valuable for:

Condition	Suggested Dosage
Stress/Depression	50–300 mg
Water retention	50–300 mg of vitamin B_6

Toxicity and Adverse Effects   No known toxicity and no known adverse effects are associated with this dosage of B vitamins.

Vitamin C (Ascorbic Acid)

Vitamin C is probably the most popular and widely used vitamin—and with good reason. Aside from its justifiably acclaimed role in preventing or combating colds, and in general immune building, vitamin C is an antioxidant. This means that it helps to protect the body against the damage of *free radicals*. Free radicals are chemical, not political. They are atoms that join to bodily compounds, causing oxidative stress and damage. Long-term oxidative stress has been associated with signs of aging, as well as many degenerative diseases. Vitamin C and other antioxidants (like vitamin E and selenium) intercept free radicals before they can do any harm.

This means that aside from building your immune system and protecting you against the colds and flulike viruses of winter, vitamin C has a powerful antiaging effect. It also protects against cardiovascular disease by helping to prevent hypertension (high blood pressure) and atherosclerosis (hardening of the arteries that often leads to heart attacks and strokes). Vitamin C has been linked with high levels of HDL ("good") cholesterol and low levels of LDL ("bad") cholesterol.

If you are concerned about osteoporosis, you should make sure you get sufficient quantities of vitamin C. It has been associated with the formation of a bodily substance called *hyaluronic acid*. This compound is critical for maintaining healthy bones and preventing them from becoming brittle. It is also necessary for maintaining healthy connective tissue.

Supplements   Vitamin C supplements are available both as ascorbic acid and as mineral ascorbates. You should be aware that the vitamin C in most commercial supplements has been synthesized from natural, inexpensive substances such as starch, molasses, or sago palm. "Natural" vitamin C found in supplements is extracted from rose hips, which contain 1 percent ascorbic acid. Even rose hips–based vitamin C supplements contain large quantities of synthetic vitamin C, because a supplement made entirely from rose hips would be enormous in size and very expensive. However, rose hips probably contain complementary substances that enhance the absorption of the vitamin, so there may be some advantage to taking supplements that contain them. I recommend that you buy ascorbic acid supplements that contain bioflavonoids (see page 92), because these substances have been shown to increase vitamin C absorption.

Buffered vitamin C is helpful for people who suffer from stomach acid or diarrhea. Generally, the ascorbic acid has been mixed with minerals to form mineral ascorbates that protect the stomach lining from some of the erosive effects of the acid.

It is wise to avoid chewable vitamin C tablets because they are high in sugar, and the acid may cause the pH of your saliva to fall so low that calcium is leached from your tooth enamel. The same is true of ascorbic acid powder.

Recommended Dosage   For optimum general health, the basic Optimum Daily Intake for vitamin C is:

500–5,000 mg

Based on a thorough scientific review of vitamin C, and on my clinical experience, the following amounts of vitamin C appear to be valuable for:

Condition	Suggested Dosage
Coronary heart disease prevention	500–4,000 mg
High levels of stress	1,000–5,000 mg
Osteoporosis	1,000–4,000 mg
Arthritis	2,000–4,000 mg

Toxicity and Adverse Effects   There is no proven toxicity for vitamin C. If you have a history of kidney problems, you should take vitamin C only under the guidance and supervision of a qualified professional. With alterations in kidney function, the mechanism that handles vitamin C excretion may not be working, so caution is warranted. Contrary to some popular misconceptions, studies do not support a relationship between vitamin C and the formation of kidney stones in otherwise healthy individuals.

One common adverse effect of taking very high doses of vitamin C—5,000 milligrams or more daily—is intestinal gas and loose stools. Vitamin C may affect the gastrointestinal tract, so if you have a history of hyperacidity, take only buffered vitamin C, and be sure to take it on a full stomach.

Vitamin D

Vitamin D is extremely important to our health throughout our lives, and especially as we age. To be precise, vitamin D is actually not a "vitamin" at all. Rather, it is a hormone. It exerts hormonelike effects on mineral ab-sorption, bone mineralization, and certain secretions. Our bodies manu-facture vitamin D in response to sunlight. Additionally, vitamin D is present in fish liver oils and egg yolks.

Vitamin D deficiency has been associated with osteoporosis. It is par-ticularly important that postmenopausal women take regular vitamin D supplements, especially if their diet is deficient in seafood and fish. Indi-viduals with osteoporosis who have not responded to calcium supple-mentation may be advised to add moderate vitamin D and magnesium to the daily regimen, and to increase sunlight exposure.

Supplements   There are two forms of vitamin D supplements available: vitamin D_2 (ergocalciferol) and D_3 (cholecalciferol). Vitamin D_3 is the preferred form, since it is the naturally occurring form. But both D_3 and D_2 become the active hormone we call "vitamin D" after passing through the liver and kidneys.

Vitamin D is available in capsule and gel cap form, and in cod-liver oil.

Recommended Dosage   For optimum general health, the basic Opti-mum Daily Intake for vitamin D is:

400–800 IU

Based on a thorough scientific review of vitamin D, and on my clinical experience, the following amounts of Vitamin D may appear to be valu-able for:

Condition	Suggested Dosage
High blood pressure	400–800 IU
Osteoporosis	400–800 IU

Toxicity and Adverse Effects   According to several studies, amounts of up to 1,000 international units per day of vitamin D appear to be safe for adults. However, it is generally considered unwise to exceed this dosage. Symptoms of too much vitamin D are nausea, loss of appetite, headache, di-arrhea, fatigue, and restlessness. Mild cases of hypervitaminosis—a condi-tion caused by vitamin overdose—are treatable. Extended doses of over 1,000 international units can cause hypercalcemia (high levels of blood calcium) which can, in turn, lead to calcium deposits in soft tissues such as those of the kidneys, heart, lungs, and veins. These deposits may be irreversible.

Vitamin E

Like vitamin C, vitamin E is an antioxidant and it is second to vitamin C in popularity—with good reason. Vitamin E is helpful in enhancing an array of different bodily systems, including the immune and the nervous systems. It is particularly important in the battle against cancer and cardiovascular disease. It has yielded positive results in treating circulatory problems such as angina, atherosclerosis, and thrombophlebitis. Like vitamin C, it increases desirable HDL cholesterol levels, and lowers undesirable LDL cholesterol levels. It is useful in wound healing, and is commonly prescribed to lessen the risk of internal scar formation in women who have had breast implants following breast cancer.

Vitamin E plays a vital role in the prevention of age-related degenerative diseases. It actually seems to slow the aging process itself. Furthermore, it delays the onset of menopause and reduces the number and intensity of hot flashes once the menopausal changes are under way. Once you are past the menopause itself and are struggling with age-related skin problems, you will find vitamin E to be helpful in combating vaginal dryness and general skin dryness. Brown "age spots" will respond nicely to topical as well as oral vitamin E supplementation.

The best news of all: Vitamin E has been shown to be highly effective in combating hot flashes. Combined with herbs and soy isoflavones, it is a powerful anti–hot flash formula.

Supplements　Vitamin E actually consists of eight substances, of which alpha-, beta-, delta-, and gamma-tocopherol are the most active. There are natural and synthetic forms of all the tocopherols. The naturally occurring form of vitamin E is the "D" form, as in D-alpha tocopherol. The synthetic form is the "DL" form, which contains only a small proportion of natural vitamin E. The natural form appears to be the most absorbable.

Vitamin E supplements often contain alpha-tocopherols alone, because that has been shown to be the most active form. However, many nutritionists recommend that you buy "mixed" tocopherols, since that is how they exist in food.

Vitamin E is measured in international units (IUs) or milligrams (mgs). One milligram is equal to approximately 1.5 international units.

Recommended Dosage   For optimum general health, the basic Optimum Daily Intake for vitamin E is:

400–1,200 IU

Based on a thorough scientific review of vitamin E, and on my clinical experience, the following amounts of vitamin E appear to be valuable for:

Condition	Suggested Dosage
Aging	400–800 IU
Cardiovascular disease prevention	400–800 IU
Hot flashes	400–1,200 IU
Poor circulation	600–1,200 IU

Toxicity and Adverse Effects   If you have high blood pressure, you should not take large amounts of vitamin E (over 400 international units) unless you are being monitored by a professional. If you are taking blood pressure medication, you may need to have the dosage adjusted, because vitamin E may actually lower your blood pressure. In addition, you should start with a low dose of 200 international units and increase it gradually. If you are taking anticoagulants, do not take large amounts of vitamin E (above 400 international units) without professional supervision.

Taking less than 800 to 1,200 international units of vitamin E appears to be safe and free of toxicity. However, *very* high doses—over 1,200 international units per day—can cause nausea, flatulence, diarrhea, headache, heart palpitations, and fainting. These are very rare and completely reversible when the dosage is decreased.

Minerals for Menopause

Minerals are inorganic elements, meaning that they are not produced by plants and animals. Like vitamins, they function as coenzymes, enabling chemical reactions to occur throughout the body.

Minerals belong to two groups: the *macro* minerals that require higher intakes; and the *micro* minerals that should be taken in smaller, trace amounts. The macro minerals include calcium, magnesium, and phosphorus. The micro minerals—also called trace minerals—include zinc, iron, copper, manganese, chromium, selenium, iodine, potassium, and boron. Minerals are stored in various parts of the body—primarily in bone and muscle tissue. Therefore it is possible to overdose on minerals if you take extremely large amounts.

Calcium

Our bodies contain approximately 1,200 grams—about 2.5 pounds—of calcium. Almost all of it is stored in our bones and teeth, although some of it is distributed throughout the rest of our bodies.

Calcium is one of the most important minerals for everyone, and especially for postmenopausal women. Correct levels of calcium in the body will protect against hypertension. Some studies have even suggested that it can be more effective than antihypertension drugs in lowering high blood pressure. It's also free of the unpleasant side effects so frequently associated with antihypertensive drug treatment, such as fatigue, weight gain, dizziness, and impaired concentration.

Calcium is used by the body to activate the enzymes involved in fat and protein digestion, and in the production of energy. It is involved in blood clotting and the transmission of nerve impulses. It aids in the contraction and expansion of the muscles, including the heart, and in the absorption of many important nutrients—especially vitamin B_{12}.

The most important reason for postmenopausal women to focus on calcium is that it is such an essential mineral for bone health. In the average adult, about 600 to 700 milligrams of calcium are exchanged in the bones every day. Normally, if there is sufficient calcium being absorbed from the diet, the blood and bone calcium levels stay in balance and fluctuate only slightly. However, if the diet is deficient in calcium, the body will always choose to maintain a certain level of calcium in the blood by drawing it out of the bones. From the body's point of view, it is more important to maintain minimum blood levels of calcium so as to keep the heart beating regularly than it is to keep the bones strong and hard.

The process of calcium reintegration into bone tissue is accomplished through a complex set of chemical interactions involving numerous hormones, and other compounds, including vitamin D. In fact, even if there is enough calcium in the diet, a lack of vitamin D will seriously impair the body's ability to make use of the mineral. If too much calcium is removed from the bones, osteoporosis sets in.

Postmenopausal women are especially vulnerable to calcium depletion because estrogen is one of the hormones involved in sustaining mineral levels in the bones. As estrogen levels drop, calcium can be leached from the bones at a more rapid pace than it is replaced. So it is crucial that postmenopausal women get enough calcium in their diets, adding supplements when necessary.

Supplements Calcium supplements are available as tablets, as flavored chewable squares, and in liquid form. The supplements generally combine pure, or "elemental," calcium with other chemicals, or "salts." The forms most commonly available are calcium aspartate, calcium carbonate, calcium citrate, calcium gluconage, and calcium lactate. When buying calcium supplements, be sure to consider the amount of *elemental* calcium rather than the amount of calcium salts. (The package should give you this information.) Of the various forms available, calcium carbonate contains the greatest amount of elemental calcium—40 percent. Many people prefer this form because the higher calcium content allows them to take fewer pills to obtain their Optimum Daily Intake. Calcium carbonate and calcium lactate are both quite absorbable, but calcium citrate is probably the most absorbable for older individuals. This is because with advancing age, the stomach reduces its output of hydrochloric acid. Calcium citrate requires little hydrochloric acid for absorption.

I generally advise that calcium supplements be taken along with magnesium and vitamin D, since these three nutrients work together to enhance one another's absorption and utilization in the body. Also, taking calcium supplements without magnesium may result in magnesium deficiency—a deficiency that has been implicated in osteoporosis. The calcium-to-magnesium ratio should be approximately 2 to 1. Fortunately, there are now many supplements that contain a proper balance of these two minerals. Some even have additional vitamin D.

Dolomite is a supplement that contains both calcium and magnesium. However, because this product contains these minerals in their least absorbable form, I don't recommend its use. Bone meal, another source of calcium, is absorbable; however, it contains substantial amounts of phosphorus. Most people get more than enough phosphorus in their diets.

Finally: Many antacids are being promoted as calcium supplements, since these products contain calcium carbonate. However, some also contain aluminum, a toxic mineral that actually interferes with calcium absorption, and can have many other deleterious effects on the body. If you choose to use antacids as a source of calcium supplementation, be sure to read the label carefully and check that aluminum is not an ingredient.

Recommended Dosage   For optimum general health, the basic Optimum Daily Intake for calcium is:

500–1,000 mg

Based on a thorough scientific review of calcium, and on my clinical experience, the following amounts of calcium appear to be valuable for:

Condition	Suggested Dosage
Broken bones/Fractures	1,000–2,000 mg
High blood pressure	1,000–1,500 mg
Osteoporosis	1,200–2,000 mg

Since the body cannot absorb 1,000 milligrams all at once, divide your doses into halves or thirds, and take them two to three times a day. Make sure to take calcium in combination with magnesium (in a ratio of 2 to 1), and with vitamin D.

Toxicity and Adverse Effects   Calcium has no known toxic effects. A panel of the Food and Drug Administration (FDA) concluded that calcium intakes of 1,000 to 2,500 milligrams daily do not result in hypercalcemia—excessively high levels of calcium in the blood. Although hypercalcemia may be seen in certain medical conditions, and in cases of vitamin D overdose, a high intake of calcium is not in itself the causative factor. The development of kidney stones in connection with high calcium intake is rare.

Some people report a feeling of relaxation and drowsiness after taking calcium supplements. This has never been documented in a scientific study. However, if you experience this particular effect, enjoy it! Schedule your calcium supplements in the evening before retiring.

Chromium

The adult body contains approximately 6 grams of chromium. The highest concentrations of this mineral are found in the hair, spleen, and kidneys. The heart, pancreas, lungs, and brain also contain this trace mineral, but in lower concentrations.

Chromium's primary role in the body is to activate enzymes involved in the metabolism of sugar and the synthesis of proteins. If you suffer from any sugar-related disorder—such as diabetes or hypoglycemia—chromium will be an extremely helpful supplement. Chromium supplements, coupled with a diet and exercise program, have enabled some of my diabetic patients (both insulin- and noninsulin-dependent) to reduce their insulin injections or discontinue their oral medications.

Chromium deficiency has also been implicated in high cholesterol levels that place people at risk of atherosclerosis (hardening of the arteries). Chromium supplements increase high-density lipoproteins (the HDLs, or "good" cholesterol) and decrease low-density lipoproteins (LDLs, or "bad" cholesterol) in addition to lowering overall cholesterol levels. It is therefore a valuable tool in the fight against cardiovascular disease.

Here's some additional good news: Chromium might be helpful in increasing lean body mass (muscle) and reducing the percentage of body fat. Used responsibly, Chromium supplementation may help you in the perennial "battle of the bulge."

Supplements   Chromium is available as an individual supplement, and as a component of some multivitamin-mineral formulas. It is produced in several forms, including chromium chloride, GTF (glucose tolerance factor) chromium, chromium polynicotinate, chromium dinicotinate, and chromium picolinate (probably the most commonly available form). All these forms are effective. In my clinical practice, I have found that individuals respond differently to the various types of chromium. Therefore, if you don't achieve the desired results with one supplement, you should try another form.

Recommended Dosage   For optimum general health, the basic Optimum Daily Intake for chromium is:

200–600 mcg

Based on a thorough scientific review of chromium, and on my clinical experience, the following amounts of chromium appear to be valuable for:

Condition	Suggested Dosage
Diabetes	400–600 mcg
High cholesterol, high LDLs, low HDLs	400–600 mcg
Hypoglycemia	200–600 mcg
Impaired glucose tolerance	400–600 mcg
Weight loss	400–600 mcg

Toxicity and Adverse Effects   There is no known toxicity for chromium, except in the cases of chromium mining and industrial exposure, which cause chromium dust to be inhaled.

Copper

The body contains about 100 to 150 milligrams of copper, stored in the liver, brain, heart, and kidneys. Copper is also found in the hair.

Copper helps your body absorb and use iron to synthesize *hemoglobin*—the stuff that makes your blood red. It also is important for your nerves, your taste sensitivity, and your connective tissue, bones, and skin. It helps combat many inflammatory diseases, including rheumatoid arthritis, osteoarthritis, and sciatica. Copper-containing drugs are often used in the treatment of ulcers, convulsions, cancer, and diabetes. It is thought that copper facilitates the tissue-repair processes that use copper-dependent enzymes.

Supplements   Copper is available as an individual supplement and is often included in multivitamin-multimineral supplements as well. The most common available forms of this supplement are copper gluconate and copper sulfate. Copper citrate is also available. I generally recommend copper gluconate, as it is gentler to the digestive tract. However, when taken in amounts as small as 2 milligrams, any of these forms may be well tolerated.

Recommended Dosage   For optimum general health, the basic Optimum Daily Intake of copper is:

0.5–2 mg

There is not enough data to permit me to make recommendations for specific conditions and concerns at this time. I recommend using a zinc-to-copper ratio ranging from 10 to 1, to 15 to 1. Copper and zinc will work well together and potentize each other in these proportions.

Toxicity and Adverse Effects   If you suffer from Wilson's disease, you should avoid taking copper. In Wilson's disease, copper accumulates in the liver and is then released and absorbed by other parts of the body, causing toxicity. The symptoms of this condition include hepatitis, degeneration of the lens of the eye, kidney malfunction, and neurological disorders. Extremely high doses of copper can produce nausea, vomiting, abdominal pain, diarrhea, headache, dizziness, and a metallic taste in the mouth. If untreated, this can lead to death.

Iron

Every cell in the body contains and requires iron, a mineral essential for all physical functions. The most important use of iron is in transporting oxygen. This is accomplished through the hemoglobin in our red blood cells. Iron is also present in a variety of enzymes and plays a key role in keeping our immune system healthy. People who are iron-deficient are usually *anemic*. They are pale, listless, cold, weak, and often suffer from headaches.

Women are particularly vulnerable to anemia because they lose blood every month through their menstrual cycles. During perimenopause, while you are still menstruating, you must be especially vigilant about your iron levels. It is easy to dismiss fatigue and mood swings as just "part of the change" when in reality they may be due to iron deficiency. On the other hand, you should not assume that fatigue or constant feelings of coldness are necessarily signs of anemia and start self-medicating with supplemental iron—especially if you have no history of anemia. See your health-care provider, who will conduct an evaluation of your blood. This will determine whether or not you need additional iron.

Supplements   Iron is available as an individual supplement and as a part of many vitamin-mineral formulas. The most common form is iron sulfate, which is very inexpensive but can be irritating to the digestive tract. I generally recommend iron glycinate, iron fumarate, and iron gluconate, since they are less likely to cause constipation or other gastric disturbances. As with all other minerals, the "elemental" content is most important, so read those package labels carefully.

Recommended Dosage   For optimum general health, the basic Optimum Daily Intake for women is:

18 mg

Based on a thorough scientific review of iron, and on my clinical experience, the following amounts of iron appear to be valuable for:

Condition	Suggested Dosage
Iron-deficient anemia	25–30 mg
Poor attention span	15–20 mg

A few additional caveats about anemia: Anemia due to iron deficiency will respond fairly rapidly to supplementation. Nevertheless, supplements should be continued for several months to fully replenish the body's stores.

You should also be aware that anemia may be due to causes other than iron deficiency. These include deficiencies in vitamin B_{12} or folic acid, as well as internal bleeding. Anemia can be the side effect of several medications, as well as the result of a sports injury.

Toxicity and Adverse Effects   The body has a highly effective mechanism that prevents iron overload and toxicity. Consequently, it is unlikely that you can "overdose" on iron—especially if you keep your intake below 75 milligrams per day.

Nevertheless, it is unwise to self-medicate with iron supplements, and there is no reason to do so. Your physician can order an excellent and highly reliable blood test to determine whether or not you need iron supplementation. This is extremely important, because some studies have suggested that excessive levels of iron may *increase* your risk of cardio-vascular disease. Moreover, some people suffer from a rare but dangerous condition known as hemochromatosis, which can cause the excessive absorption of iron. This results in a buildup of excess iron in the tissues and organs, and consequent damage to the liver, heart, and pancreas. This condition can be genetic, or can be acquired through excessive long-term iron intake or blood transfusions. It can easily be detected through a blood test.

Magnesium

We discussed magnesium briefly when we looked at calcium. Remember that the most important form in which magnesium is utilized by the body is in conjunction with calcium. Let's look now at some of the functions performed by this important mineral.

Magnesium is crucial to the production of enzymes and the process by which cellular energy is released. It is a powerful and very important muscle relaxant. When calcium flows into muscle tissue cells, the muscle contracts. When calcium leaves and magnesium replaces it, the muscle relaxes. Magnesium deficiency often leads to muscle spasms, tremors, and convulsions. Together with sodium, potassium, and calcium, magnesium affects the muscle tone of the blood vessels. This may help to explain why magnesium supplementation helps control cardiovascular disease.

Magnesium plays an important role in bone growth and helps prevent tooth decay by holding calcium in tooth enamel. Poor magnesium intake has been implicated in disorders such as osteoporosis.

Recommended Dosage   For optimum health, the basic Optimum Daily Intake for magnesium is:

500–750 mg

Based on a thorough scientific review of magnesium, and on my clinical experience, the following amounts of magnesium appear to be valuable for:

Condition	Suggested Dosage
Angina	500–1,000 mg
High blood pressure	500–750 mg
Osteoporosis	500–1,000 mg

Toxicity and Adverse Effects   Magnesium toxicity is rare, except in individuals with kidney disease. In healthy individuals, large quantities of magnesium salts—3,000 to 5,000 milligrams daily—have a cathartic effect, and magnesium-containing products are often used as over-the-counter laxatives.

Manganese

Manganese is an important mineral, but is used only in tiny quantities by the body—just about 10 to 20 milligrams are present at any given time. Minuscule but powerful, manganese is involved in various enzyme systems. It works with dozens of different enzymes that facilitate processes throughout the body, including protein, fat, and carbohydrate metabolism. Manganese helps to maintain proper functioning of the nervous and the immune systems, and also helps in the metabolism of sugar.

Most important for our purposes, manganese helps repair bones and connective tissue and maintain bone density in postmenopausal women.

Recommended Dosage   For osteoporosis or various forms of arthritis, the recommended dose is 15 to 30 milligrams daily.

Toxicity and Adverse Effects   Manganese is safe and nontoxic when it is ingested in the form of either manganese-rich foods or supplements. Serious brain damage can occur, however, when manganese is inhaled (as in the case of certain miners who are exposed to high concentrations of manganese oxide in the air) or when it is drunk in large quantities in manganese-contaminated well water.

Potassium

Our cells contain more potassium than any other mineral. A total of approximately 250 grams of this nutrient can be found in the adult body.

A growing body of evidence indicates that low levels of potassium are associated with high blood pressure—an association that is particularly high when the sodium-to-potassium ration is high. There is also evidence to suggest that potassium helps protect the body against stroke.

Many older adults do not take in enough potassium because they are on cholesterol-reducing diets that curtail consumption of meat, dairy products, and poultry. Even patients who supplement their potassium intake with potassium-rich foods such as bananas usually do not get enough of this important mineral in their diet. All too often, these individuals are taking diuretics to control their blood pressure. The amount of potassium in food is minimal compared with the amount excreted in urine as a result of diuretic use.

Supplements Potassium is available in tablet and liquid forms. Levels above the Optimum Daily Intake should be taken only under the advice of a professional.

Recommended Dosage Under ordinary circumstances, most people do not need to take potassium supplements, because potassium is widely available in so many foods. It would be better to reduce sodium intake so that a sodium-to-potassium ratio of 1 to 1 is achieved. If, however, you are taking diuretics, lowering your blood pressure, or are concerned about your potassium, you can take:

99–300 mg

Toxicity and Adverse Effects Potassium toxicity is seen when daily intakes exceed 18 grams, an amount that is unlikely to be ingested through food. Toxicity usually occurs only through the uneducated use of supplements, or when an individual is experiencing kidney failure. Excess potassium may cause muscle fatigue, irregular heartbeat, and possibly heart failure.

Selenium

Selenium, a trace mineral, is present in all tissues of the body but is concentrated most highly in the kidneys, liver, spleen, and pancreas. Many

Americans suffer from selenium deficiency because our diets are typically low in selenium-containing foods, and because the soil in which our food is grown is usually low in this mineral.

Selenium is an important antioxidant, protecting us against the damages brought about by the unchecked action of free radicals in our bodies. Proper selenium intake helps combat degenerative diseases, as well as cancer. Additionally, selenium helps to protect against cardiovascular disease, to stabilize mood, and to minimize the toxic effects of mercury, arsenic, and excessively high levels of copper.

For perimenopausal and postmenopausal women, selenium is particularly important because it has a positive effect on the skin and mucous membranes. It can help to keep your body skin, as well as your vaginal lining, healthy, supple, and elastic.

Recommended Dosage   For optimum health, the basic Optimum Daily Intake for selenium is:

100–200 mcg

Based on a thorough scientific review of selenium, and on my clinical experience, the following amounts of selenium appear to be valuable for:

Condition	Suggested Dosage
Arthritis	100–200 mcg
Heart disease	100–200 mcg

Toxicity and Adverse Effects   A human being must consume vast quantities of selenium for toxicity to become a problem. It is generally thought that overt selenium toxicity may occur if 2,400 to 3,000 of selenium are ingested daily. Toxicity symptoms include a garlic odor in the breath, urine, and sweat.

Zinc

Our bodies contain a relatively large quantity of zinc—approximately 2 to 3 grams. Distributed throughout the body, zinc is an essential building block of over twenty enzymes associated with a wide array of different metabolic processes.

Zinc plays a critical role in cell division, cell repair, and cell growth. It is essential for maintaining good vision and protecting against cataract formation, optic neuritis (the inflammation of the optic nerve), and night blindness. If you enjoy the aroma of a rose or if you savor the tang of an apple, you can thank zinc, which plays an important part in your senses of smell and taste. Zinc is helpful to the immune system and is widely recommended as a supplement if you are fighting off a cold.

Postmenopausal women should be aware that zinc is important in maintaining hormonal balance and also in keeping the bones, teeth, and hair strong.

Supplements   Zinc is available as individual supplements and as part of many multivitamins and multimineral formulas. In supplements, pure or "elemental" zinc is combined with other compounds. Of these, I feel that zinc gluconate and zinc citrate, which are sometimes referred to as chelated zinc, are probably the best choices for most people. They are relatively inexpensive and well tolerated. While zinc sulfate is also inexpensive, it is irritating to the stomach. Many practitioners use other forms of zinc, such as zinc picolinate and zinc orotate, because they believe that these are the most absorbable forms. Unfortunately, there is no convincing data to support these claims.

Since zinc supplements combine elemental or pure zinc with another compound, when buying supplements you must consider the amount of elemental zinc, which is commonly listed on the product label.

Recommended Dosage   For optimum general health, the basic Optimum Daily Intake for zinc is:

22.5–50 mg

Toxicity and Adverse Effects   The symptoms of zinc toxicity are gastrointestinal irritation and vomiting. Zinc is actually recognized as an emetic—a substance that induces vomiting. However, this form of toxicity occurs only when 2,000 milligrams or more have been ingested. There is also some evidence linking long-term excessive zinc intake (more than 50 milligrams a day) to copper deficiency.

Essential Fatty Acids

We have already discussed essential fatty acids (EFAs) extensively in chapter 3 (pages 32–63), so we will not belabor the subject here. I'd ask you to refer to that discussion. You can certainly get much of your Optimum Daily EFA requirements through the dietary suggestions I outlined.

Many people, however, do not get enough EFAs in their diet. Making the transition to a diet high in fish, borage, flaxseed, and black current oils can be challenging and difficult to orchestrate. Moreover, many factors can interfere with the conversion and absorption process of EFAs. These include smoking, environmental toxins, aging, excessive saturated fat intake, alcohol, and certain medications. Supplements provide you with preformed, already-converted, instantaneously usable EFAs.

This section will detail the various EFA supplements—which particular EFA will help your perimenopausal and postmenopausal symptoms or conditions, in what form the supplement is available, and how much you should take. The table on pages 122–23 will assist you in matching EFAs to your specific set of symptoms.

Omega-3 Fatty Acids

The two most important omega-3 fatty acids are eicosapentaenoic acid (EPA) and docosahexaenoic acid (DHA). These are available in the form of fish oil supplements. In general, each fish oil tablet contains between 180 and 400 milligrams of EPA, plus 120 to 300 milligrams of DHA. Although cod-liver oil contains EPA and DHA, large doses should be avoided, because the oil also contains high amounts of vitamins A and D, which—if ingested in very large quantities—could be toxic.

Make sure your EPA and DHA supplements include vitamin E to prevent rancidity, and that you take additional vitamin E to prevent oxidation in the body. While there is no Optimum Daily Intake, most studies have used eighteen or more fish-oil capsules without controlling dietary fat intake. You can achieve the same clinical benefits by eating a low-fat diet and using smaller amounts (four to six capsules). Because of this nutrient's blood-thinning effect, higher amounts should be taken only under professional supervision, especially if you are also taking blood-thinning medication.

Omega-6 Fatty Acids

The omega-6 fatty acid most needed by the body is called gamma-linolenic acid (GLA). While it is present in most vegetable oils, the body's ability to convert the plant components into usable GLA is often inhibited by environmental and other factors. The vegetable oils that contain more potent and accessible GLA—such as borage and black currant oils—are generally not used in cooking. For this reason, GLA supplementation is extremely important.

Both in scientific studies and in clinical practice, capsules of evening primrose oil have been the mainstay of GLA supplementation. The problem is that each evening primrose capsule contains only 45 milligrams of GLA along with over 100 milligrams of linoleic acid—the EFA that has inflammatory effects. For this reason, borage and black currant oils are more effective. Each capsule of borage or black currant oil contains 240 to 300 milligrams. I generally recommend 240 milligrams of GLA (1 capsule) daily. Higher amounts should be taken only under professional supervision, so as to avoid upsetting the fatty acid balance in your body.

Which Fatty Acids Should You Take?

How do you know whether to supplement with omega-3 or omega 6? Or both? After all, the omega-3 and the omega-6 fatty acids do overlap to a great degree and some confusion as to which one to take is natural. The truth is that EFA supplementation isn't an exact science. Often, it is a case of trial and error. As a general rule of thumb, I tend to use EPA when there is a family tendency of high cholesterol (170 or above), high triglycerides, heart arrhythmias, or other heart disease. For those with low cholesterol, I generally use GLA. For menopausal problems, I usually try GLA first. However, keep in mind that researchers and clinicians have observed individual responses to the different fatty acids, so you must be willing to experiment. Try one type of supplement for one month, and then switch to the other. Compare the results and stick with whichever one is most effective. If the results are not clear-cut, you may have to use both to achieve the balance that is right for you. In fact, some practitioners suggest giving EPA/DHA and GLA supplements together, and studies have shown that EPA and GLA used together yield the best results for some purposes, such as decreasing the inflammation of rheumatoid arthritis.

Other Nutritional Supplements

Our bodies require many different kinds of nutrients other than vitamins, minerals, and EFAs. Some—such as acidophilus—replace bodily compounds destroyed by such medications as antibiotics. Others—such as kelp—help to combat the negative effects of environmental pollutants. Still others are rich in phytoestrogens and help in restoring hormonal balance during the menopausal years.

Acidophilus

For the digestive tract to successfully carry out the myriad chemical changes involved in digestion, several important substances must be present. One of these is called *Lactobacillus acidophilus,* or just acidophilus for short. It is actually a bacterium, but a very friendly one. It helps to detoxify harmful substances and, paradoxically, has an antibacterial as well as an antifungal effect. When insufficient quantities of acidophilus are present, stomach gas, bloating, constipation, and malabsorption of nutrients often occur. Typically this happens after a person has completed a course of antibiotic treatment, because antibiotics destroy the "good" bacteria together with the "bad."

Acidophilus is particularly useful for women going through the menopausal transition because it prevents the reabsorption of estradiol, the form of estrogen that in high amounts is destructive to post–reproductive-age women. Its presence in the gut allows the body to dispose of this estrogen before it can circulate and bind to estrogen receptors in the breast, leading to breast cancer. It also can help prevent urinary tract infections and vaginal yeast infections—two common conditions that often affect postmenopausal women as the linings of their urinary tract and vagina become thinner, less supple, and more vulnerable.

Supplements   You can obtain acidophilus at your health food store. It is available in powder as well as capsule form. The most common strain of this friendly bacterium is called *lactobacillus acidophilus,* although some supplements contain several different strains, including *bifidobacteria.* The best supplements are those that contain more than one strain of acidophilus, and that require refrigeration. While there are some strains that can survive at room temperature, the freshest and most effective products need to be refrigerated.

Recommended Dosage   Since different supplements provide varying amounts of acidophilus, it is difficult to come up with a single recommended dosage. There are no hard-and-fast rules covering acidophilus supplementation. My advice is to follow directions on the label.

Toxicity and Adverse Effects   There is no known toxicity or any adverse effect associated with acidophilus.

Coenzyme Q_{10}

Coenzyme Q_{10} is also known as *ubiquinone,* because it is ubiquitous—it exists everywhere in the body. Like other enzymes, coenzyme Q_{10} (also known as CoQ_{10}) is a catalyst. It plays a crucial role in energy production because it catalyzes the chain of chemical reactions that create *adenosine triphosphate* (ATP), a compound that yields energy needed by cells to function. CoQ_{10} is also an important antioxidant that scavenges harmful free radicals, thereby preventing cell damage.

$CoQ_{10}$is a powerful asset in the battle against cardiovascular disease. Studies have found it to be particularly effective in the treatment of angina. It has also been proven effective in reducing the amount of tissue damage that occurs during open-heart surgery or a heart attack. CoQ_{10} helps to regulate arrhythmia (irregular heartbeat), and may also help in the treatment of other heart problems. Finally, CoQ_{10} protects low-density lipoproteins (LDLs, or "bad" cholesterol) from oxidation and lowers overall elevated serum cholesterol. It also raises high-density lipoproteins—HDLs. Often called the "good" cholesterol, a high HDL level protects against heart disease.

You can help protect your gums against the ravages of periodontal disease with CoQ_{10} supplementation. You can also strengthen your muscles. This, in turn, will have a positive impact upon your bones.

Recent studies have shown that very large amounts of CoQ_{10} can be effective therapy for women with late-stage breast cancer.

Supplements CoQ_{10} is generally available in 10-, 30-, 50-, 60-, 100-, and 120-milligram capsules.

Recommended Dosage There is no Optimum Daily Intake for CoQ_{10}. Generally, 50 to 300 milligrams have been used in clinical trials, and appear to be safe and effective. Some trials have used as much as 600 milligrams, but this higher dose should be used only under the guidance of a professional. I usually recommend 100-200 mg as a basic daily dose— which will also be especially helpful for breast cancer prevention. If you already have breast cancer, I urge you to work with a competent health-care professional to ascertain the best dosage for your particular condition.

Toxicity and Adverse Effects CoQ_{10} appears to have very few adverse effects, although there have been some reports of gastrointestinal upset, loss of appetite, nausea, and diarrhea associated with very high doses.

DHEA

DHEA, which stands for dehydroepiandrosterone, is one of the five major sex steroid hormones that we touched upon in chapter 2. Produced by the adrenal glands, it is central to the regulation of the body's response to stress. It is also converted to other hormones, such as estrogen, progesterone, and testosterone.

Natural DHEA is available at health food stores. This leads many unsuspecting women to believe that they can take it without medical guidance if they suspect that they may be suffering from DHEA deficiency. But this is not a safe practice. Self-medicating with DHEA can be a serious mistake! You should use DHEA supplementation under the supervision of your physician or health-care provider, who will order a salivary hormone test to determine whether you are indeed deficient in this particular hormone. And since DHEA affects the levels of other hormones in your system, all your hormonal blood or saliva levels should be monitored regularly.

Supplements DHEA is available in tablet, capsule, and liquid form.

Recommended Dosage The usual dosage of DHEA is 10–50 milligrams per day. Some practitioners recommend that it be taken all at one time; others recommend divided doses. Consult your health-care provider for the form and dosage most suited to your needs.

Toxicity and Adverse Effects   Hormone supplementation should never be undertaken without the supervision of your health-care provider, because it must be monitored carefully and regularly. DHEA is the precursor to both estrogen and testosterone, so adverse effects can occur if an overdose of DHEA leads to elevation of one of these hormones.

Flavonoids

Flavonoids (also called "bioflavonoids") are crystalline compounds found in plants. Since the first flavonoid was identified in 1936 by the Nobel Prize–winning scientist Albert Szent-Gyorgy, scientists have isolated more than four thousand flavonoids. Yet even this large number may represent only a small fraction of all the flavonoids that exist in nature.

Flavonoids give plant foods much of their color and zest. They are responsible for the beautiful deep color in berries and are also found in citrus skins, vegetables, nuts, seeds, grains, legumes, tea, coffee, cocoa, and wine. Most medicinal herbs owe their therapeutic qualities to flavonoid compounds.

Flavonoids are important antioxidants—possibly more powerful than vitamins C and E. They possess antiviral, anticarcinogenic, anti-inflammatory, and antihistamine qualities, and also offer important protection against cardiovascular disease.

The phytoestrogens we discussed in chapter 3 comprise one particular class of flavonoids. I hope that, as you incorporate the dietary suggestions included in that chapter into your lifestyle, you will be consuming increasingly large quantities of phytoestrogens through such foods as soy and legumes. If, however, your diet is deficient in these important plant compounds, you can take several important supplements.

Supplements and Recommended Dosage   I would counsel you to go to the health food store and browse through the shelves of soy supplements. Study the labels carefully, because you want to know the amount of soy isoflavones in the product. I generally recommend that you have at least one 50-to-100-milligram serving of soy isoflavones each day. Soy protein drinks, for example, contain very high concentrations of isoflavones, while some brands of "soymilk"—a tasty substitute for dairy—contain almost none at all.

Toxicity and Adverse Effects   No known toxicity of soy has been reported. A few cases of *hyperestrogenism* (high levels of estrogen) have been reported in women consuming massive doses of soy—generally over 100 grams per day. The Food and Drug Administration (FDA) recommends 25 grams of soy protein each day to reduce the risk of heart disease and lower serum cholesterol. This level of intake has been shown to be completely safe and effective.

Gamma-Oryzanol

This extract of rice bran oil is a side-effect-free supplement that has been associated with relief of perimenopausal complaints such as hot flashes, insomnia, headaches, depression, and anxiety. One study showed that 85 percent of the participants experienced marked relief of many of these symptoms. These results have been replicated in other studies as well.

Supplements   Gamma-oryzanol is available in tablet, capsules, and softgel form.

Recommended Dosage   The recommended dosage of gamma-oryzanol is 100 mg, three times daily. The most effective way to take it is together with vitamin E, and many supplements—called E-gamma-oryzanol—have already combined them for you.

Toxicity and Adverse Effects   No known toxicity or adverse effects are associated with gamma-oryzanol.

Ipriflavone

Ipriflavone is an isoflavone that is synthesized from daidzien—one of the most important phytoestrogens found in soy products. Although it is a relative newcomer to the American menopausal supplement armamentarium, numerous studies have already supported its effectiveness in combating osteoporosis.

Ipriflavone inhibits bone resorption and increases the absorption of calcium by the bones. In other words, it prevents calcium from being lost and helps it to be acquired and incorporated into bone tissue. Conventional drug therapy is classified as being either antiresorptive or bone-forming. Ipriflavone is both.

Ipriflavone should be used preventively by women with a family history of osteoporosis. It is also an effective treatment for those already diagnosed with the disease. In fact, studies have shown it to be not only comparable but actually superior to estrogen replacement in its ability to increase bone density.

Supplements   Ipriflavone is available in tablet and capsule form. It can be found, too, in bone-building products that also provide bone-strengthening minerals such as calcium and magnesium.

Recommended Dosage   The recommended dosage is 600–1,200 mg daily.

Toxicity and Adverse Effects   Long-term studies of human beings, as well as extensive study of animals, have shown that ipriflavone is quite safe. The most common side effects reported are gastrointestinal. These disappear when the dosage is reduced.

Kelp

Kelp is a type of seaweed. Most of us have grown up associating seaweed with the stuff we pick from between our toes at the beach, but many seaweeds are actually quite high in all sorts of nutrients. They form an important part of the diet in other cultures.

Kelp is a rich source of vitamins, minerals, and many trace elements. In fact, it contains fifty-six mineral and trace elements. Studies have shown that some of the ingredients in kelp help to counteract the adverse effects of radiation, heavy metals, and other environmental toxins. Kelp has also been associated with increased digestive, endocrine, cardiovascular, immune, and nervous health. It is rich in iodine, which is essential for keeping your thyroid gland healthy. It may also be helpful to those who suffer from thyroid problems. Daily intake of kelp can help to heal disorders of the gastrointestinal tract—such as ulcers. Its strong and unusual taste makes it an interesting addition to your cooking, and it is often used as a salt substitute for those who must restrict their salt intake.

Kelp has particular relevance to women going through the menopausal transition. Studies have shown that it can prevent or reduce fibrocystic breast tissue, ovarian cysts, uterine fibroids, menstrual cramps, and hot flashes. Its high mineral content helps to prevent osteoporosis as well.

Supplements   While kelp can be eaten raw, it is also available in dried, granulated, or powdered form. If you do not like the taste, you can purchase tablets at the health food store.

Recommended Dosage   All kelp supplements list the iodine content on the package. The recommended therapeutic dosage is 150–300 mg of iodine daily. If you are using kelp in your cooking, you can reduce or eliminate additional kelp supplementation.

Toxicity and Adverse Effects   Kelp itself is without adverse effects. However, because our oceans have become so polluted, it is important that you check your sea vegetables to make sure they are clear of toxins. While currently no federally approved organic certification or quality-control standards exist for sea products, you can cut down on contaminants in your sea vegetables by carefully reading the packaging to determine if the producer is concerned about processing and pollution.

Herbal Supplements: Self-Standing Herbs

Herbal therapy—also called *phytotherapy,* or plant therapy—is a more gentle, natural approach to perimenopausal and postmenopausal symptoms than conventional prescription or over-the-counter medications. Of course, many conventional medications are derived from plants. In fact, the word *drug* comes from the Dutch word *drogge,* which means "to dry out," because the leaves and roots of herbal plants had to be dried out and usually ground before they could be used medicinally. The difference between herbs and conventional medicines concerns the degree to which the products are refined, processed, and combined with other constituents that are synthetic or animal based.

There are many wonderful herbs that can help you with perimenopausal discomforts and postmenopausal conditions. This section will introduce you to the most useful and easy-to-obtain herbs that can address the most common complaints. These are the "front line" herbs—the most popular, basic herbs that address perimenopausal or postmenopausal complaints. These are also the herbs that have received the most scientific attention and validation. You will learn the name (common and botanical) of each herb, which part of the plant is used, what symptom or condition the herb addresses, what dosage should be taken, and how the herb should be used. The next section will focus on herbal combinations—herbs that work best when taken together. Tables 4.1 on page 122 and 4.2 on page 124 will provide you with a step-by-step guide to herbal supplementation during menopause.

As a rule, you will not use herbs the same way you would use vitamins and minerals, and other nutritional supplements. Since most Americans—women as well as men—have diets that are woefully insufficient in basic nutrients, supplements such as vitamins and minerals are important, whatever your age, gender, or circumstances. There is an Optimum Daily Requirement for each nutrient—a minimum quantity necessary to maintain good health. If you suffer from a given ailment, you can increase your intake of a particular vitamin, mineral, or other nutritional supplement in order to address the condition in question, but a certain baseline minimum must be taken in at all times.

This is not the case with herbs. There is no Optimum Daily Requirement that, if you dip below it, will result in compromised health and well-being. Herbs are used exclusively to address symptoms or give added support to an already-healthy system. Tonic herbs and adaptogens, for example, help an otherwise-healthy body adapt to stressful times and circumstances. Most other herbs are used medicinally—to rectify systemic imbalances, bring about symptomatic relief, or cure illness. So in the sections below, you will not find a recommended dosage for general use, only recommendations designed to remedy specific conditions.

Buying and Storing Herbs

You can obtain herbs at a health food store. An increasing number of supermarkets and pharmacies are beginning to carry them as well. While herbs are available in a variety of forms—dried roots, stems, or leaves which can be purchased by the pound; teas; decoctions; and tinctures—I will concentrate here only on prepackaged herbs. Most of these are standardized and are manufactured by major and reliable herbal companies. These are available in capsule, tablet, or liquid form with dosages clearly marked on the label.

The government has taken a strange and equivocal stance toward herbs. They are seen as "nutritional supplements" rather than medications and are not subject to regulation. There is no quality control. For this reason, it is hard to know whether the product you are buying actually contains the product it is supposed to contain, and in quantities that are pure and therapeutically helpful. So make sure you look for a brand that says "standardized" and gives quantities on the label. Ginseng, for example, should say "standardized to 5 percent ginsenosides." Otherwise, you may not actually be getting the product you think you are getting. The substance you have taken won't be effective, and you will walk away discouraged, saying that "herbal medicine doesn't work."

Herbs should be stored in a cool, dry place. Like vitamins, they should not be kept in the refrigerator, or on top of it. An ordinary kitchen cabinet should be more than sufficient.

Black Cohosh (*Cimecifuga racemosa*)

Black cohosh is probably the most popular and widely used menopausal herb, both in Europe and in the United States. If you were going to start with a single herb to address a wide range of the most common complaints, I couldn't recommend one more highly. It has ancient origins and uses, as well as modern scientific substantiation—truly the best of both worlds. Native Americans, who called it "squaw root," used it extensively in treating a variety of female disorders, including premenstrual discomforts, pregnancy-related pain and distress, and postpartum disorders. They also used it to address premenstrual discomforts. Black cohosh has been used extensively since the early 1940s in Germany as a natural hormonal agent for treating premenstrual and perimenopausal symptoms. Today, black cohosh is the most well-researched and scientifically supported herbal remedy for the entire range of menopausal symptoms.

Symptoms Addressed The effectiveness of black cohosh in treating perimenopausal complaints has been substantiated by numerous scientific studies. It has been proven effective in addressing and remedying the most common discomforts—hot flashes, fatigue, irritability, night sweats, headaches, and insomnia. Additionally, it has a stabilizing effect on blood pressure, rectifying hypotension as well as hypertension, and decreasing heart palpitations.

Supplements   Black cohosh is available in the form of tablets or capsules. The most reliable brand—and the one that has been most widely studied by scientists in Germany—is called *Remifemin®*. American companies, however, do manufacture black cohosh supplements, either self-standing or in combination with other helpful herbs.

Recommended Dosage
1–2 tablets per day

Toxicity and Adverse Effects   There are no known contraindications or adverse effects associated with black cohosh. The German E Commission—the world's most respected and accepted scientific authority on herbs—recommends the herb's use for six months, although no evidence of toxicity or side effects has ever been reported in women. Historically, black cohosh has been used for longer periods of time.

Some women report mild, transient stomach upset when they first begin using the herb.

Chaste Berry (*Vitex agnus castus*)

Like black cohosh, chaste berry has a long history, dating back to ancient times. In ancient Greece, it was considered to be a protection against dangers and also connoted chastity. In fact, according to Greek mythology, the goddess Hera—who was regarded as the protectress of marriage—was born under a Vitex bush. The word *castus*—Latin for "chaste"—continued the connotation of chastity through medieval times, when chaste berry was considered to be a suppressor of libido.

Today we know that this herb does not have a negative impact on libido. It *does* support normal menstrual and reproductive functions, healthy skin, and normal functioning of the pituitary gland. Most important for our purposes, it has a positive impact on mood during perimenopause.

Symptoms Addressed   Clinical studies have verified that chaste berry balances the estrogen-progesterone levels in the body, helping to normalize the hormonal instabilities that so often lead to mood swings. If you suffer from irritability, depression, or both—either simultaneously or sequentially—chaste berry will help to stabilize your mood and help you through the emotional roller-coaster effect of perimenopause. Chaste berry also can bring relief of hot flashes.

Supplements   Chaste berry is available in liquid or capsule form. Each should provide 30 to 40 mg of the herb.

Recommended Dosage   Based on my scientific research as well as my clinical experience, the recommended dosage for chaste berry is:

40 drops of liquid extract per day

or

1–2 capsules per day

Toxicity and Adverse Effects   In general, chaste berry is considered to be safe and free of negative side effects. It occasionally causes nausea, diarrhea, weight gain, headaches, and allergic rash. These are rare and disappear when the herb is discontinued.

Garlic (*Allium sativum*)

Garlic is probably the most versatile herb. Used extensively for both medicinal and culinary purposes, garlic has received a considerable amount of attention on the part of the scientific community. This is because scientists discovered that societies and ethnic groups that consume large quantities of garlic on a regular basis—such as people living in Mediterranean countries—suffer from less cardiovascular disease.

Numerous scientific studies have borne out this association. Garlic is known to be a blood thinner. By reducing the blood's "gluey" consistency, garlic helps prevent the formation of life-threatening blood clots and of the plaque that forms along the arteries, causing atherosclerosis and leading to strokes and heart attacks. Garlic improves blood cholesterol levels by lowering LDL ("bad") and raising HDL ("good") cholesterol levels. It also helps lower potentially detrimental blood fats called triglycerides.

In addition to its cardiovascular benefits, garlic has been shown to build immunity against illness, fight colds and viruses, and even prevent cancer.

Symptoms Addressed   Because cardiovascular disease is such an important concern for postmenopausal women, garlic is a particularly important herb to incorporate into the daily routine. If heart disease runs in your family, I would urge you to begin a serious program of garlic supplementation. You would also be well advised to take garlic after meals in which you have consumed a large quantity of fat. Studies have shown that individuals who eat garlic together with saturated-fat items such as butter or steak have cholesterol counts considerably lower than those who eat the fat without the garlic. Incorporating garlic into your routine means that when you do splurge, you will suffer fewer ill effects.

Supplements   You can certainly cook with garlic, but most of the health benefits are lost through excessive cooking. Moreover, many people avoid eating garlic because of its offensive odor.

My advice is that you obtain liquid or capsules containing odorless garlic from the health food store. Because these are deodorized and specially coated, you can obtain all the health benefits without fear of becoming a social outcast. Garlic preparations are available as liquid extracts, oil-filled capsules, and tablets. The supplements generally contain 100 to 300 milligrams in each pill.

Recommended Dosage   There is no Optimum Daily Intake for garlic. If you can eat or cook with several cloves of garlic per day without ruining your social life, that's more than sufficient. If you choose to use supplements (most of which are odor modified) then you must read packages carefully. Potencies differ from product to product, and the brand you are buying will recommend a daily dosage.

Toxicity and Adverse Effects   Some people have experienced toxic reactions when taking over ten raw cloves of garlic a day. If you cook with garlic, you may experience some skin irritation from cutting too much raw garlic. A pair of rubber gloves should solve that problem.

There doesn't appear to be any adverse effect from supplementation with six capsules per day. In some people, fats in the blood may initially rise during garlic supplementation, and then begin to drop. No adverse effects have been noted as a result of this transient rise, even among heart disease patients. Higher doses could cause a sudden drop in blood pressure, and so should be taken under professional supervision only. You should also consult your health-care provider before starting garlic supplementation if you are using a blood thinner. Finally, some people may experience skin eruptions with higher doses, but this side effect subsides when supplementation is reduced or stopped.

Ginkgo (*Ginkgo biloba*)

Ginkgo has an interesting history. Among the oldest living species currently known to scientists, it has often been called a "living fossil." It apparently flourished in large forests over 150 million years ago, almost became extinct during the last Ice Age, then slowly made a resurgence in China and other parts of Asia. Due to deforestation, ginkgo went through a second near-extinction. Today, it is preserved for its medicinal and ornamental uses.

Ginkgo has numerous uses and enjoys worldwide popularity as a botanical medicine. In Germany it is one of the most popular single herbs recommended by physicians. In the United States, it recently stepped into the herbal spotlight due to heavy media coverage of a 1999 study supporting ginkgo's use in the treatment of Alzheimer's disease.

Ginkgo's positive effects are broad and far-reaching. It serves as a powerful antioxidant, as well as an anti-inflammatory herb. It is helpful for people with allergies, tinnitus (ringing in the ears), hearing loss, heart disease, stroke, memory impairment, mental confusion, and impaired vision. It improves memory and cognitive functions in the elderly and may improve venous circulation in the arms and legs.

Symptoms Addressed   Ginkgo can help perimenopausal women with fatigue, depression, and memory problems. It can help postmenopausal women who suffer from circulatory, visual, or cognitive difficulties.

Supplements   Ginkgo is available in capsule and tablet form. Look for a brand that is standardized to 24 percent ginkgo biloba content.

Recommended Dosage   For maintenance of general good health, and to address specific symptoms, the recommended dosage of ginkgo is:
120–240 mg (2 to 4 capsules) per day

Toxicity and Adverse Effects   There are no reported contraindications or adverse side effects.

Ginseng—American, Asian, and Siberian (*Panax quinquefolius, Panax ginseng, Eleutherococcus senticosus*)

There are three kinds of ginseng: Asian (Chinese or Korean), American, and Siberian. The first two are authentic ginseng. They belong to the

Panax family and are closely related species, similar in chemical constituents, pharmacological activities, and therapeutic applications. The third—Siberian ginseng—is actually not ginseng at all. Its technical name is *eleuthero*. Because it looks somewhat like the other forms of ginseng and has similar effects on the body, it is commonly called "ginseng."

All forms of ginseng are *adaptogens*. They help people adapt to changes—both internal and external—that stress the body. Revered by the ancient Chinese as well as the ancient Native Americans, ginseng has a wide range of bodybuilding applications. These include improving mental and physical endurance, strengthening the body's natural immunity, alleviating fatigue, promoting general feelings of well-being, improving memory and learning capacity, and enhancing work performance. Ginseng is replete with phytohormones and is beneficial in addressing menopausal symptoms.

Symptoms Addressed   The physical changes that take place during the perimenopausal and postmenopausal years are very stressful to the body. Ginseng helps the body to adapt to these stresses and their resultant symptoms, such as fatigue, loss of libido, and depression. Ginseng also is beneficial to the vaginal lining and alleviates some of the dryness commonly associated with menopause.

Additionally, ginseng has direct estrogenic effects. In fact, a recent case history reported a postmenopausal woman who, upon beginning ginseng treatment, began to menstruate again! Unlike ERT, however, daily ginseng use has been associated with reduced risk of most types of cancer.

Supplements   Panax ginseng products are generally standardized to 5 to 10 percent ginsenosides and are available in liquid extract, capsule, and tablet form. The label directions should tell you how much ginseng is in each unit.

Recommended Dosage   To address menopausal symptoms and to promote general feelings of energy and well-being, the recommended daily dosage of ginseng is:

200–400 mg/day

Toxicity and Adverse Effects   Ginseng should be avoided by asthmatics and emphysema patients. Allergy to ginseng is unusual, but when it occurs, it results in insomnia, pruritis, and heart palpitations. Ginseng overdose many cause similar symptoms, as well as nervousness, diarrhea, menopausal bleeding, and hypertony (increased pressure in the eyes).

Do not take ginseng together with caffeinated products.

Kava Kava (*Piper methysticum*)

Kava kava, native to Asian countries and Australia, has been used in religious ceremonies for centuries. It induces a state of mild intoxication somewhat similar to the pleasant feelings induced by marijuana or alcohol, but without interfering with cognition, sound judgment, or concentration.

When used in religious ceremonies, kava can produce effects that are more profoundly euphoriant, almost bordering on the hallucinogenic. However, the kava used by native peoples in their rituals is prepared quite differently from the kava that is used medicinally.

Symptoms Addressed   Kava is used primarily to alleviate anxiety and to help insomniacs relax and fall asleep. It can also be useful in the relief of muscular tension and achy joints due to arthritis or rheumatism. Additionally, kava is a mild painkiller, particularly effective in addressing toothaches.

Supplements   Kava is available in liquid extract and capsule form. Look for a brand that is standardized to 30 percent kavalactones.

Recommended Dosage
50–100 mg 4 times per day

Toxicity and Adverse Effects   If you are using kava in large quantities and are uninterested in sex, don't blame your partner! Regular use can lead to diminished libido. Excessive consumption of kava can also have mood-altering effects. Do not drive or operate heavy machinery under those circumstances.

St. John's Wort (*Hypericum perforatum*)

St. John's wort got its name from the religious legends associated with it. From ancient through medieval times, it was reputed to protect against evil spirits and demonic possession. Today's herbalists, who do not look upon emotional or mental disorders as signs of demonic possession or divine disfavor, regard St. John's wort as a powerful antidepressant. Numerous scientific studies have confirmed its efficacy in addressing emotional and psychological disorders—most notably depression.

Additionally, St. John's wort is a helpful diuretic and is also useful in treating neuralgic conditions such as sciatica and hip pain.

Symptoms Addressed   Depression is a common perimenopausal and postmenopausal symptom, both because of the biochemical changes occurring in the body and because of the psychosocial changes associated with the transition into and through midlife. Numerous scientific studies have shown St. John's wort to be as effective as Prozac and other antidepressants in addressing this often-debilitating condition.

Supplements   St. John's wort is available in liquid extract, tablet, and capsule form. It is important that you check the label to make sure the product has been standardized to .3 percent hypericin.

Recommended Dosage

Mild to moderate depression	900 mg per day
Severe depression	1,800 mg per day

Toxicity and Adverse Effects   The safety and lack of significant side effects have been demonstrated in human clinical trials examining the antidepressant effect of St. John's wort. Some patients have reported gastrointestinal irritations, allergic reactions, tiredness, and restlessness. If you are already taking an antidepressant such as Prozac, you should consult a competent health-care professional before starting a course of St. John's wort treatment.

Herbal Supplements: Herbs to Be Used in Combination

As a scientist, I am usually wary of recommending or using a medicinal substance that has not been backed up by rigorous scientific research. The self-standing herbs recommended in the section above—black cohosh, chaste berry, ginseng, ginkgo, kava, and St. John's wort—have all received a great deal of thorough and impeccable scientific scrutiny that substantiates their effectiveness and safety.

Scientific study is undoubtedly the gold standard of reliability, but the absence of such study does not necessarily invalidate remedies that people have used for centuries with success. Every culture has its own set of traditional herbal remedies for maintaining health and addressing illness. Research studies are not always available to support the effectiveness of some of these herbs because modern science is only at the beginning of the process of subjecting ancient herbs to modern scientific analysis. It will take a long time before the vast number of herbs known to various cultures in all parts of the world become properly researched and substantiated.

In the absence of double-blind, placebo-controlled studies of some of these herbal combinations, anecdotal evidence and history must support their use. Most of these herbs have been taken for thousands of years with excellent results and few, if any, negative effects. What's more, I have seen in my clinical practice how effective they can be in addressing menopausal complaints. My patients have experienced a great deal of symptomatic relief from the herbs described in this section.

Choosing an Herbal Formula

The herbs described below generally work more effectively as a team than alone. Some, like Don Quai, may even be useless if taken as a self-standing remedy. You can obtain prepackaged groups of herbs at the health food store. Unless you are going to consult a professional herbalist who will create a combination of herbs tailor-made to your particular set of needs, you will need to rely upon herbal manufacturers who have already assembled several herbs into a single formula designed to address an array of common menopausal symptoms.

The section below is designed to teach you a little bit about each herb, and also about which herbs work best in combination. That way, when you are staring at the health food store shelf, confronted by a bewildering and often overwhelming array of herbal products with names like "Women's Formula" or "Menopausal Relief," you will have some idea of which herbs address your discomforts and concerns. Since herbs have medicinal properties, label directions should be followed for the products you choose to take.

Cayenne (*Capsicum frutescens*)

Cayenne has culinary as well as medicinal applications. The main ingredient of chili, it adds spice and color to many dishes.

Cayenne has numerous and varied health-producing properties. It is a general stimulant, often used to build up the immune system at the onset of a cold. A catalyst for other herbs, cayenne improves circulation, aids digestion, and stops bleeding from ulcers. It has a salutary effect on the kidneys, lungs, spleen, pancreas, heart, and stomach and is said to be effective in combating nausea, rheumatism, arthritis, and pleurisy.

Symptoms Addressed   Cayenne doesn't just stimulate the digestion. It serves as a stimulant for the entire system. It is an excellent herb to use when your primary symptom is fatigue. It's also an effective remedy against weight gain, since it stimulates the metabolism.

Toxicity and Adverse Effects   Excessive consumption of cayenne can cause heartburn and stomach upset. Cayenne should be used in combination with other herbs rather than alone.

Chamomile (*Chamomilla recutita*)

Chamomile, an ancient herb, was so revered by the Egyptians for its ability to cure malarial symptoms that they dedicated the plant to their impressive pantheon of gods. Europeans have used it as a remedy for neuralgia, back pain, rheumatism, and insomnia. It is one of the most commonly found herbal teas, often served as a caffeine-free substitute for after-dinner coffee or as a mild sedative.

Symptoms Addressed   You can try some chamomile tea if you find yourself tense or anxious. You don't need tablets or liquid extracts; a simple cup of tea, perhaps flavored with lemon, will be soothing and may help you through a rough moment of your day.

Toxicity and Adverse Effects   Avoid chamomile if you are allergic to ragweed.

Cornsilk (*Zea mays*)

The delightful threads found between the husk and the kernels of fresh corn are called cornsilk. They contain many medicinal compounds and are particularly helpful for people needing a diuretic.

Symptoms Addressed Cornsilk is helpful if you suffer from hypertension or fluid retention. It can also relieve the discomfort of breast and abdominal bloating.

Toxicity and Adverse Effects There is no known toxicity associated with cornsilk. If you are allergic to corn, however, you should look for an herbal combination containing other diuretics.

Damiana (*Tumor aphrodisiac*)

Damiana has been regarded as an aphrodisiac for men as well as women. In fact, it is commonly used as part of an array of herbs to treat male impotence. It has laxative as well as generally health-building, tonic effects. Damiana is a pituitary gland regulator.

Symptoms Addressed Damiana is an antidepressant. It is also useful for stimulating libido, therefore quite helpful if you are experiencing sexual difficulties. Since people who are depressed often experience loss of libido, and sexual difficulties often contribute to depression, damiana is an excellent herb to help break that vicious cycle.

Toxicity and Adverse Effects If you are using a formula that contains damiana and it has not alleviated your symptoms within a few weeks, then switch to another formula containing other herbs that will address depression and loss of libido.

Dandelion (*Taxacum officinale*)

Many of us work very hard to eliminate the bright yellow flowers that dot our backyards. Because dandelions are regarded as weeds and have such a poor reputation among gardeners, some of us have grown up believing that they are poisonous. That isn't true. Dandelion is an important herb and has been used for centuries as a diuretic and a digestive aid. It has also been used to address high blood pressure, anemia, and jaundice.

Symptoms Addressed Formulas containing dandelion will help you if you are experiencing constipation, are bloated, or suffer from hypertension. Additionally, if you are still menstruating and your flow has become heavier than it used to be, you will need to guard against iron-deficiency anemia. Dandelion will help you to do this.

Toxicity and Adverse Effects There is no known toxicity, and no adverse effects are associated with dandelion.

Don Quai (*Angelica sinesis*)

Not to be confused with its cousin Angelica—an herb commonly used to address respiratory complaints—this fragrant, perennial herb grows in Mainland China, Korea, and Japan. Its strong aroma is an interesting blend of celery and licorice. Its use in Asia as a menopausal remedy dates back to ancient times. It was introduced into Western medicine in 1988 by Merck (of *Merck Manual* fame) in the form of a liquid extract sold under the name of *eumenol* and recommended for the treatment of menstrual disorders.

Symptoms Addressed Don Quai is particularly helpful in addressing hot flashes, irritability, insomnia, restlessness, night sweats, and headaches.

Toxicity and Adverse Effects Do not use herbal formulas containing Don Quai during your menstrual period if you suffer from hypermenorrhea (excessive bleeding during menstruation). Don Quai is most effective when used in combination with other herbs rather than alone.

Gentian (*Gentiana lutea*)

Commonly known as bitterroot or bitterwort, gentian is a herbaceous perennial plant found in Europe and Asia Minor. It has been cultivated in the United States as well. It's a pretty plant, sporting large, bright yellow flowers that bloom during the summer months.

For centuries, herbalists in Europe, China, and India have used it to treat a variety of digestive complaints. Gentian addresses digestive problems by stimulating gastric secretions. It also stimulates the appetite—something to watch out for if you tend to have a problem with overeating. It is good for liver and spleen function, fever, colds, and gout.

Symptoms Addressed   If you suffer from digestive disturbances—nausea, vomiting, or diarrhea—associated with hormonal fluctuations, an herbal combination containing gentian would be particularly helpful for you.

Toxicity and Adverse Effects   There is no known toxicity associated with gentian.

Gotu kola *(Centella asiatica)*

Gotu kola, a low-growing herb with heart-shaped leaves, originates in India, where it has been used for centuries as a brain tonic. Ancient yogis used it to calm the mind prior to meditation. It also contains compounds that promote tissue healing, improve circulation, and improve memory. Studies have linked gotu kola with improvement of varicose veins.

Symptoms Addressed   Gotu kola is helpful in addressing emotional symptoms associated with menopause—irritability, anxiety, and also depression. It has both a stimulating and a calming effect on the nerves. If memory loss is a significant problem for you, then look for an herbal combination containing gotu kola. Varicose veins also respond nicely to this herb.

Studies have shown that gotu kola is most potent when combined with ginkgo biloba, so look for an herbal combination containing both of them.

Toxicity and Adverse Effects   There is no known toxicity associated with gotu kola.

Hops *(Humulus lupulus)*

Although the hop vine can be found in many parts of the world, it is cultivated primarily in the United States. The unusual name *hops* applies to the scaly, conelike fruit that develops from the flowers.

Hops has all sorts of varied and interesting applications. It is good for nervousness, restlessness, pain, stress, and insomnia. It has been used successfully to diminish the desire for alcohol and to improve circulation. It stimulates the appetite, dispels flatulence, and relieves intestinal cramps and spasmodic coughing. Hops has diuretic properties as well.

Hops can be used externally in a very unusual way. Folk wisdom suggests stuffing a pillow with hops that has been lightly sprinkled with alcohol as a remedy for insomnia.

Symptoms Addressed   If you suffer from nervous discomforts, such as irritability, restlessness, and insomnia, hops will be very effective—especially if combined with valerian. Bloating and fluid retention will also respond well to hops.

Toxicity and Adverse Effects   Hops is very safe with extremely low toxicity.

Juniper Berry (*Juniperus communis*)

A sixteenth-century Dutch pharmacist soaked the dark purple berries of the evergreen juniper shrub in distilled alcohol and offered them to the public as a new drug. Its medicinal properties were rapidly overshadowed by its recreational qualities, and soon people on the Continent as well as in England were drinking it as an alcoholic beverage, which English-speaking people called *gin*.

Juniper relieves inflammation, flatulence, and sinusitis. It helps in the treatment of pancreas, kidney, and bladder problems. It is useful to diabetics because it regulates blood sugar levels. It is also an effective diuretic.

Symptoms Addressed   Juniper is helpful if you are experiencing fluid retention—breast or abdominal bloating—or general edema.

Toxicity and Adverse Effects   Juniper berry is very safe with extremely low toxicity. Overdoses may be harmful to the kidneys.

Licorice (*Glycyrrhiza glabra*)

Licorice, a popular candy, is also a powerful herb with a three-thousand-year history of use as a medicinal plant. In the ancient worlds of Greece and

China, licorice was used to treat respiratory symptoms as well as gastrointestinal disorders. Hippocrates used it as a topical ointment, Napoleon used it as an antacid, and the Dutch physician E. F. Revers used it during World War II for soldiers suffering from indigestion.

Symptoms Addressed   Licorice has anti-inflammatory, antibacterial, immune-enhancing, and expectorant qualities. In addition, it raises energy levels by stimulating the adrenal glands. The Chinese regard it as a strengthener of *qi,* the vital life force.

Licorice appears to lower estradiol levels while raising progesterone levels. It helps reduce a broad range of menopausal symptoms, including hot flashes and fatigue.

Toxicity and Adverse Effects   People with kidney problems, high blood pressure, or hypokalemia (an abnormally low concentration of potassium in the blood) should check with their physicians before taking licorice, since high doses may raise blood pressure. High doses are not recommended for individuals who must adhere to a low-salt regimen or individuals taking diuretics, corticoid treatments, cardiac glycosides, or medications for hypertension.

Licorice root is generally safe and very effective when used in combination with other herbs.

Red Clover (*Trifolium pratense*)

Red clover is a legume widely used by farmers as a crop to improve soil quality. Most scientific research has concentrated on its agricultural effectiveness, and the two studies exploring its effectiveness as a menopausal remedy were inconclusive. It is very popular, however—especially in Australia—and there is a substantial amount of anecdotal evidence to support its use.

Symptoms Addressed   Red clover addresses ovarian symptoms, such as ovarian cysts. It stimulates the ovaries to maximize estrogen production—even during perimenopause, when estrogen production is dropping. For this reason, it is often helpful in alleviating hot flashes.

Toxicity and Adverse Effects There is no known toxicity, and no adverse effects are associated with red clover.

Red Raspberry (*Rubus ideaus*)

Many of us have gone raspberry picking during the summer and have enjoyed the sweet, juicy red fruits that stained our fingers and made delicious jam. Raspberries have medicinal as well as culinary applications and have been used for centuries by women to address an array of reproductive conditions and disorders. These include morning sickness, menstrual cramps, and menopausal discomforts.

Symptoms Addressed Raspberry helps tone weak uterine muscles and relaxes uterine and intestinal spasms. Rich in phytoestrogens, it helps maintain hormonal balance and reduce discomforts—such as hot flashes—that arise from hormonal imbalance. If you suffer from a prolapsed uterus—a condition in which the uterus slips out of place and rests on the bladder, causing urinary incontinence and generalized discomfort—raspberry can help to correct this structural condition.

Toxicity and Adverse Effects There is no known toxicity, and no adverse reactions are associated with red raspberry.

Sage (*Salvia officinalis*)

Sage has a history dating back to medieval times. It was reputed to be a powerful, almost panacealike herb. In fact, its botanical name, *Salvia,* comes from the Latin verb *salvere,* which means "to save."

Sage was used to treat tuberculosis patients suffering from night sweats, to address gum disease, and to relieve gastrointestinal discomforts such as stomach cramps and flatulence.

Symptoms Addressed Because sage has antiperspiration qualities, it is particularly useful in addressing hot flashes and night sweats.

Toxicity and Adverse Effects There is no known toxicity, and no adverse effects are associated with sage.

Sarsaparilla (*Similax officinalis*)

Sarsaparilla originally hails from the American tropics. It was brought to Europe by Spanish traders in the 1600s, where it was regarded with a certain amount of awe. It was used to treat syphilis, promote urination and sweating, and remedy impotence in men. Applied externally, sarsaparilla was also used to address parasitic conditions, such as ringworm.

Symptoms Addressed   Sarsaparilla is particularly helpful for perimenopausal and postmenopausal women who are experiencing diminished libido and energy levels. Because this herb stimulates testosterone production, it boosts sexual as well as general physical energy.

Toxicity and Adverse Effects   There is no known toxicity, and no adverse effects are associated with sarsaparilla.

Shepherd's Purse (*Capsella bursa-pastoris*)

This herb, sometimes called pickpocket and St. James's weed, is a common and virtually ubiquitous plant. It is sturdy enough to make its appearance in meadows, fields, along roadsides, and in junkyards. Believe it or not, it has important medicinal properties. Shepherd's purse is a diuretic and a coagulant, quite effective in addressing excessive internal or external bleeding. Because it has a constricting effect on muscles, it has also been used to promote uterine contractions during childbirth. It can help constipation by promoting intestinal contractions and stimulating the production of a bowel movement.

Symptoms Addressed   For perimenopausal women, shepherd's purse is helpful because of its ability to normalize progesterone levels. If you are approaching menopause and your menstrual periods are excessive, or have become irregular, this herb will help you to regulate and increase the length of your cycle until the natural cessation of the menses.

Toxicity and Adverse Effects   There is no known toxicity, and no adverse effects are associated with shepherd's purse.

Uva Ursi (*Arctostaphylos uva ursi*)

Uva ursi's folk name is bearberry. This herb has been used since ancient times as a folk remedy for urinary tract infections. Modern scientific research has substantiated this traditional use, supporting its effectiveness for the treatment of bladder and kidney ailments. Some people have also found it to be an effective remedy for hemorrhoids.

Symptoms Addressed   If you suffer from bloating due to fluid retention—either in your abdomen or in your breasts—then look for an herbal combination containing uva ursi. It is an excellent and highly effective diuretic. It is also an appropriate herb to take if you are experiencing urinary tract difficulties.

Toxicity and Adverse Effects   There is no known toxicity, and no adverse effects are associated with uva ursi.

Valerian (*Valeriana officinalis*)

Although valerian has a name similar to Valium and has often been called the "Valium of the nineteenth century," this herb is chemically unrelated to the real Valium. It is a relaxant, commonly used to treat anxiety. It is highly effective in the treatment of panic attacks, irritability, and stress-induced insomnia. Additional uses include the treatment of ulcers, headaches, colic, gas, muscle cramps, and circulatory disorders. Some people have found valerian helpful in reducing mucus production during a cold or the flu.

Symptoms Addressed   If you suffer from anxiety, irritability, insomnia, or nervous tension, valerian would be an essential remedy to try. It has no negative effects, nor does it interact poorly with medications or alcohol as some of the prescription antianxiety medications (such as Valium and Xanax) do. A powerful muscle relaxant, valerian may also be helpful in relieving menstrual cramps.

Toxicity and Adverse Effects   There is no known toxicity, and no adverse effects are associated with valerian.

Wild Yam (*Dioscarea villosa*)

Wild yam has become quite popular in addressing menopausal complaints and has been the subject of some noteworthy studies. It is a perennial vine that grows in a variety of North American regions, including the Northeast, the Southeast, Texas, and Minnesota. Wild yam was used by Native American women for birth control and to prevent miscarriage. It is used by today's pharmaceutical companies to synthesize oral contraceptives. It has also been used for a variety of nonmenopausal purposes, since it has antispasmodic, anti-inflammatory, diuretic, antiemetic, and expectorant effects. It is said to be soothing to the nerves.

There is a great deal of confusion surrounding wild yam, and many different wild yam products are available on the market. You can obtain several different oral preparations. While self-standing tablets are available, most oral wild yam products combine several different herbs that work more efficaciously together than alone.

One of the most popular—and confusing—forms of wild yam is the topical creams. There are two different kinds of topical wild yam creams on the market. While both are made from wild yams, they are actually quite different. One type of cream contains nothing but natural wild yam, sometimes mixed with other herbs. The other contains laboratory-manufactured progesterone, which has been chemically processed from wild yams. Both creams are available over the counter.

Using wild yam creams to address progesterone imbalance should not be undertaken without professional guidance. We will return to this subject in chapter 7 when we discuss natural hormone replacement.

Symptoms Addressed   Since wild yam has strong estrogenic as well as progestogenic properties, it serves as an excellent force to balance erratic hormones. It may reduce heavy bleeding or regulate the unpredictable spotting and staining that often accompany the menopausal transition. Its anti-inflammatory effects can be quite helpful in addressing the occasional joint pain that some women experience during perimenopause.

Recommended Dosage   Since each product is different, you will need to follow directions on the label.

Toxicity and Adverse Effects   Adverse effects may occur if you use wild yam cream that contains progesterone, and it elevates your progesterone levels above normal. Again, it is essential to undertake hormone supplementation—even "natural" hormones—under the guidance and supervision of a health-care professional.

Ayurvedic and Chinese Herbal Combinations

There are literally hundreds of herbs that hail from the Indian and the Chinese traditions, and dozens of formulas. Seeking the advice of a practitioner of these disciplines will help assure that your specific symptoms are addressed. However, if you want to explore Ayurvedic or Chinese herbal remedies on your own, here are a few tips.

Ayurvedic Herbal Combinations

Ayurveda means the "science of life" in Sanskrit. This ancient Indian system of healing dates back well over five thousand years. It was first developed by the *Rishis* (holy men) who believed that a healthy body would better enable them to pursue their spiritual goals.

In general, Ayurveda focuses on maintaining health, although it also addresses specific illnesses. Its teachings differ from our Western concepts of illness and health. Ayurvedic healers have a complex set of categories by which they classify human beings. Each person is a unique blend of the five elements of life (earth, fire, water, air, and ether), classified into three main groups, called *doshas*. The doshas include *Vata* (ether and air), *Pitta* (fire and water), and *Kapha* (earth and water). Healing is based on balancing these doshas through proper diet, spiritual and emotional balance, and herbal medicines.

There are several important herbs that Ayurvedic healers use to address menopausal complaints. If you visit a healer in person, he or she will take an extensive history, study your own unique physiological and psychological profile, and recommend a combination of herbs specifically suited to your needs. If you wish, however, you can try to self-medicate with some of the most common herbal combinations—such as those listed below—that an Ayurvedic physician would employ. These products are available at your health food store. You can also order them directly from the manufacturer.

Based on my research as well as my clinical experience, I advise my patients to try the Ayurvedic formulas listed below.

- **MenoCare:** An herbal blend developed to address estrogen and progesterone deficiencies. Use it to alleviate palpitations, insomnia, mood swings, and hot flashes.
  Dosage: 2 tablets, twice daily.

- **Geriforte:** An herbal blend developed to address the overall stress of aging. A clinical study demonstrated a reduction in most menopausal symptoms.
  Dosage: 2 tablets, twice daily.

Both of these should be available at most well-stocked health food stores. You can, however, order them directly through the manufacturer, Himalaya, USA (1-800-869-4640).

- **Midlife for Women I:** An herbal blend specifically designed for perimenopausal issues, this product helps set the stage for a healthy menopausal transition through supporting hormonal balance.
  Dosage: 1 tablet, twice daily.

- **Midlife for Women II:** These two formulas were developed to be taken together to ease women through a healthy menopause and address common menopausal symptoms such as hot flashes, mood swings, insomnia, and other symptoms associated with menopause.
  Dosage: 1 tablet twice daily, along with Midlife for Women I.

Both of these should be available at most well-stocked health food stores. You can, however, order them directly through the manufacturer, Maharishi Ayur-Ved (1-800-826-8424).

Traditional Chinese Medicine

Traditional Chinese medicine has a long and illustrious history, dating back well over four thousand years. This ancient school of medicinal thought teaches that the most important factor influencing human health is *qi* (sometimes written as *chi*), or energy flow within the body. Energy travels along specific pathways, called **meridians**. Illness is due to blocked or misdirected energy.

All Chinese menopausal herbal combinations are designed to release blocked energy and enable it to travel along correct pathways. These combinations sometimes address specific organs, as well as the overall physical balance. Menopausal formulas use herbs that strengthen female organs as well as overall energy flow.

Based on my research and my clinical experience, I advise patients to try the formulas listed below.

- **Nu Ke Ba Zhen Wan (Women's Precious Pills):** This product is an herbal combination of Rehmannia root, Don Quai root, *Codonopsis pilosula, Polia cocos, Atractylodes macrocephala, Peonia albiflora, Ligusticum wallichii,* and *Glycyrrhiza uralensis* (licorice root). It is generally used to address low estrogen levels, posthysterectomy disorders, hot flashes, forgetfulness, confusion, insomnia, and weepiness.

  You can obtain this product at health food stores or directly from the manufacturer. Manufactured by Ethical Nutrients (1-800-638-2848), it is called Eight Treasures®.

  Dosage: Take eight small pellets, three times daily. Follow label directions or advice of practitioner.

- **Hsaio Yao Wan:** This product, another ancient Chinese herbal remedy for menopause, contains *Bupleurum chinese, Paeonia lactiflora, Atractylodes chinensis, Poria cocos, Zingiber officinale* (ginger root), *Glycyrrhiza uralensis* (licorice root), and *Mentha haplocalyx* (peppermint). It will be helpful if your primary symptoms are irritability, anxiety, headaches, sugar cravings, and fatigue. It is not recommended if you are experiencing breakthrough bleeding.

  You can obtain this product at health food stores or directly from the manufacturer. Manufactured by Ethical Nutrients (1-800-638-2848), it is called Jade Empress®.

  Dosage: Take eight small pellets, three times daily. Follow label directions or advice of practitioner.

- **Liu Wei Di Huang Wan:** This herbal combination contains *Rehman-*

nia glutinosa, Dioscorea opposita (wild yam), *Comus officinalis, Paeonia suffructicosa, Poria cocos,* and *Alisma plantagoaquatica.* It is generally used as an antiaging tonic, addressing dry skin, vaginal dryness, skeletal problems, night sweats, insomnia, and loss of muscle tone.

You can obtain this product at health food stores or directly from the manufacturer. Manufactured by Ethical Nutrients (1-800-638-2848), it is called Six Immortals®.

The above Ayurvedic and Chinese formulas contain blends of herbs that have been passed down for centuries by traditional healers. Which will work best for you can be determined only by trial and error.

I have formulated my own product, called Dr. Shari Lieberman's For Women Only Advanced Changes, available exclusively through QVC, item #A45821. It is a combination of vitamins, minerals, Chinese herbal blend, black cohosh, and Vitex agnus castus.

Homeopathy and Menopause

Homeopathy is a relatively new medicinal approach. It was innovated 180 years ago by Samuel Hahnemann, a German physician. It is based on several principles, including the Law of Similars and the Law of the Infinitesimal Dose.

The Law of Similars teaches that like cures like. In fact the word *homeopathy* is derived from two Greek words—*homoios* (similar) and *pathos* (suffering). This contrasts with *allopathy,* which is the Western medical model. Allopathy teaches that a symptom should be counterbalanced and eradicated by its opposite. Stomach acid, for example, is treated by antacids that alter the pH balance of the gastric system. The runny nose of a cold is dried up with antihistamines. Homeopathic physicians, on the other hand, believe that during a cold, mucus production often is the result of the body's attempts to throw off an undesirable organism and restore physiologic balance. A homeopathic remedy might gently facilitate this response and foster drainage. Homeopathic remedies stimulate the body's own healing mechanisms instead of working against them.

According to the Law of the Infinitesimal Dose, tiny "potentized" doses of remedies matching symptom patterns stimulate the body's healing mechanisms, helping the patient to overcome the disease. These remedies become more powerful as they become more dilute, so the most infinitesimal dose is therefore the most potent. Homeopathic remedies are said to work on an energetic rather than a strictly physical level, and the more dilute the physical substance, the more powerful its energy.

The homeopathic approach to menopausal problems is that they represent imbalances that predate the onset of perimenopause and actually have been present for a long time. The remedies are designed not only to bring symptomatic relief but also to redress the physical imbalance that has spawned the symptom.

If you consult a classical homeopath, you will receive a remedy wholly suited to your particular constitutional makeup, not only your symptoms. If you wish to self-medicate, however, you can obtain individual homeopathic remedies as well as homeopathic menopausal combinations at health food stores. You will find a list of reliable homeopathic companies in the Resources section, page 201.

Homeopathic remedies should be taken fifteen minutes before or after you have eaten or brushed your teeth, and an hour before or after you have drunk coffee or some other caffeinated product. They should be stored in a cool, dry place. Because the original substance is so dilute, homeopathic remedies almost never have side effects or contraindications.

Putting It All Together

This chapter has provided you with a powerful armamentarium. You now have an array of alternative healing tools at your disposal. Tables 4:1 and 4:2 will help organize some of this material for you. They will guide you through the often-bewildering maze of supplements. Together with a healthy diet, a sensible exercise regimen, and a positive outlook, these nutritional supplements should help you to rectify imbalances and address unpleasant symptoms so that you feel healthy and energetic.

The following table is designed to help you decide which supplements to take when you are experiencing perimenopausal discomforts. But first, a few general guidelines.

- *Be sure you are taking a multivitamin-multimineral supplement.* This will supply you with basics. For many women, the addition of essential vitamins and minerals to their daily diet is sufficient to alleviate their symptoms. If yours do not abate, however, then—
- *Begin with black cohosh.* This herb is the most comprehensive available. It will address the most common symptoms—hot flashes, fatigue, irritability, night sweats, fluid retention, weight gain, and loss of libido. If your symptoms continue, then—
- *Add vitex.* This herb, together with black cohosh, forms a powerful team. These may not be enough, however. In that case—
- *Add ginseng.* In Asia, ginseng is regarded as a tonic to assist both men and women through midlife transition, and through the aging process that follows.
- *If you continue to be symptomatic,* then use the table below to match vitamins, minerals, herbs, and other nutritional supplements to your symptoms by trying a multiherb menopausal formula. Remember to find a formula that contains black cohosh, vitex, and ginseng since these are such crucial herbs, with such wide-ranging applications.

There are many formulas to choose from, so you should be able to find a product that contains several of the herbs listed below. It is unlikely, however, that you will find every herb you're looking for in a single formula. Choose your combination product on the basis of your symptoms, selecting the one that contains the most herbs to address your particular configuration of complaints.

- *Try Ayurvedic or Chinese formulas* if you have been unsuccessful with over-the-counter formulas. You might also consider experimenting with homeopathic remedies.

The word *experiment* is key. This is often a trial-and-error process. If one herb is ineffective, another might work well. Each individual responds to herbs in a unique way, based on her own unique constitutional profile. You will have to see what works best for you.

Table 4:1 Supplements for Perimenopause

Symptom	Vitamin	Mineral	Herb	Other Supplement
Hot flashes	E		Don Quai Wild yam Licorice root Raspberry Red clover	EFAs Gamma oryzanol Acidophilus
Vaginal atrophy	E		Don Quai Wild yam Licorice root Raspberry Red clover	EFAs Gamma oryzanol Acidophilus
Depression/Irritability/ Insomnia	B complex		Valerian Hops Skullcap St. John's wort Raspberry Kava kava Passion flower	EFAs
Fatigue	B_{12}	Chromium	Gotu kola Sarsaparilla Kelp	

Symptom	Vitamin	Mineral	Herb	Other Supplement
Memory loss/ Concentration	B Complex		Gentian root Cayenne Ginkgo biloba Gotu kola	
Weight gain/ Sluggish metabolism		Chromium Iodine	Gentian root Cayenne Sarsaparilla Gotu kola	Kelp EFAs
Bloating/Fluid retention	B_6 E	Magnesium	Raspberry Cayenne Gotu kola Licorice Sarsaparilla Red clover Juniper berry Uva ursi Cornsilk	EFAs Kelp
Loss of libido	E	Chromium Iodine	Damiana Vitex	Gamma oryzanol EFAs Acidophilus

Table 4:2 Supplements for the Postmenopausal Years

Many of the perimenopausal discomforts fade and eventually disappear after menopause. Some—such as vaginal atrophy and loss of libido—remain problematic and may be addressed using the supplements listed above.

You should certainly continue taking your basic multivitamin-multimineral supplement. In addition, you might want to focus on the two main concerns that arise after menopause—cardiovascular disease and osteoporosis. Here are some suggestions.

Symptom	Vitamin	Mineral	Herb	Other Supplement
Cardiovascular disease	E C	Magnesium Chromium	Garlic	Fish oil Coenzyme Q$_{10}$ EFAs Ipriflavone
Osteoporosis		Calcium Magnesium Manganese Zinc Copper Boron		
Cancer prevention	Vitamin A Beta-carotene Vitamin E Vitamin C	Selenium	Garlic Licorice Ginseng Black cohosh	EFAs

Five

Incorporating Exercise into Your Menopausal Program

The last four chapters have focused on what goes *into* your body during your perimenopausal and postmenopausal years—what you eat, what you drink, what you don't eat or drink, and what supplements you can take to ease the transition and maximize comfort. Optimal nutrition, in the form of a well-balanced diet as well as a useful array of supplements, is a central component of your menopause program.

Dietary changes and nutritional supplements, however, aren't enough to bring about optimum health at any age. Exercise is at least as important. Exercise helps your body make maximum use of the healthy foods and supplements you've been taking in. Exercise helps you metabolize your food, lose body fat, enhance immune function, increase bone density, and prevent cancer and heart disease. It also stabilizes your hormones, lifts your mood, and helps you feel generally terrific!

This chapter will take a careful look at the role of exercise at this time of your life. It will explain why exercise is beneficial to your health, what kinds of exercise—aerobic and weight bearing—are most beneficial, and how you can incorporate these exercises into your lifestyle.

Why Exercise Is Essential to Good Health

The need to "incorporate" exercise into our lives is a relatively new phenomenon. If I look at how my great-grandmother lived, for example, I see a dramatically different lifestyle. Great-grandma walked to all her destinations. When she was a child, she did not plop herself on the couch to watch television, because televisions hadn't been invented. She was either in the kitchen helping with meal preparations or outside playing. She jumped rope. She swam in the creek. She walked to and from school. She walked to her friends' houses. When she grew up and became a mother herself, she walked to the store to buy milk or bread for the family. She washed the clothes on a washing board. She got down on her hands and knees and scrubbed the floor.

Our ancestors' lives were filled with exercise. They engaged in both aerobic and strength-building exercises. Aerobic exercise consists of sustained, continuous, repetitive movements, such as brisk walking or bicycling. In aerobic exercises, you are inhaling on a regular basis and using the oxygen you've taken in to release stored energy. Strength-building exercises, on the other hand, are anaerobic. Your breath comes irregularly in gasps or spurts. Walking would be an example of an aerobic exercise, while lifting the heavy laundry basket might be an example of strength building. Great-grandma engaged in both activities every day and didn't even know the name for what she was doing! If you had told her that she was engaging in "aerobic" and "anaerobic" exercises, she would have looked at you with bewilderment and told you she was "just living."

Our lifestyle today is very different. We hop into the car to reach most of our destinations. We push a button on the washing machine or dryer. We sit in an office or stand behind a cash register, often for many hours at a time. Our bodies were not designed for this sedentary lifestyle. Study after study shows that the modern way of living, beginning with childhood and going right through our senior years, is destructive to our health. In order to offset the negative impact of the lifestyle most of us lead, we must find ways of injecting exercise into our daily (or at least our weekly) schedules.

What does exercise actually *do* for our bodies? Scientists have identified several significant areas of health that are improved by engaging in regular exercise, and are damaged when we allow ourselves to slide into a sedentary lifestyle. Let's look at what these are.

Cardiovascular Health

Exercise is one of the most powerful measures you can take to prevent and treat heart disease. Aerobic exercise is particularly effective, because it involves the continuous elevation of the pulse for a regular period of time. Aerobic exercise is associated with higher levels of protective "good" HDL cholesterol and lowers the levels of total as well as "bad" LDL cholesterol. It helps improve the circulatory system by lowering blood pressure levels. This ensures better blood flow and more efficient utilization of oxygen by the cells.

Literally hundreds of studies have focused on the beneficial impact that aerobic exercise has on cardiovascular health. Studies have shown that even people who consume large quantities of red meat, butter, and eggs often do not suffer from high cholesterol if they engage in regular aerobic exercise. They have fewer heart attacks, fewer strokes, and lower blood pressure. That doesn't mean you should discard all dietary caution! It does mean, though, that aerobic exercise is one of the most effective tools available for you to prevent cardiovascular disease, and to reverse it if you already suffer from the problem. Before you try any cholesterol-lowering medications, try this simple, noninvasive, free remedy, together with the diet program outlined in chapter 3.

Boosting Immunity and Preventing Cancer

Your immune system protects you from organisms that seek to invade your body and make themselves comfortable. Consider the immune system to be an army of cells and substances that sally forth to attack foreign and destructive invaders.

Exercise is a powerful immune-booster. Because it facilitates brisk and efficient circulation of blood, it ensures that the "soldier" cells—such as those natural killer cells that destroy viruses, bacteria, and even cancerous agents—are transported promptly to the affected area, and can rapidly vanquish invading germs. In fact, numerous studies have pointed to the role of aerobic exercise in reducing the risk of certain forms of cancer. Exercise also enhances the production of white blood cells and phagocytes, all of which are instrumental in keeping the body free from invading organisms.

Although not all the immune-boosting effects of exercise are understood, it is clear that exercise is one of the best means of supporting your immune system and fostering good health.

Stabilizing Hormonal Levels

Aerobic exercise has a generally stabilizing and balancing effect on bodily secretions and substances. Why? First, aerobic exercise burns off excess body fat, which plays a crucial role in maintaining proper hormonal balance. Stored fat cells produce estradiol—the kind of estrogen that is undesirable during the postreproductive years. Reducing body fat, on the other hand, helps reduce the amount of estradiol present in the body.

Aerobic exercise also helps your hormones circulate efficiently and rapidly by keeping the blood moving at a steady and brisk pace. Thus, hormones such as estradiol, which need to be converted into another form, are properly and speedily converted. Hormones that need to be excreted reach their destinations faster. The speed with which these processes take place means that at no time does sluggish circulation allow destructive hormones to settle in. The prompt and efficient removal of destructive hormones, and the evening out of hormonal dips and peaks, contributes to a significant reduction in perimenopausal symptoms such as hot flashes.

Preventing and Treating Diabetes

Remember what we discussed in chapter 3 about refined sugar? When you eat a chocolate bar or a slice of white toast, your blood sugar levels rise. Your pancreas works particularly hard to produce insulin that can assist in metabolizing the sugar into a form that your body can utilize, and your liver labors to store the sugar in your cells by converting it into fat. Usually, this process takes place without a problem. But if you eat too much sugar, your pancreas becomes overstressed. Eventually it may break down and stop producing enough insulin to handle the sugars—and even the complex carbohydrates—you consume. The inability of the pancreas to produce sufficient quantities of insulin is called diabetes, and it afflicts millions of Americans today.

Clearly, diet is the most important preventive measure you can take against diabetes. But diet alone isn't enough. Aerobic exercise is a crucial component of a diabetes prevention program. It burns free-floating sugars in the bloodstream, lessening the load that is placed upon the pancreas. This can actually reduce the amount of insulin you need if you are already diabetic. And because aerobic exercise lowers fat levels, it increases your body's receptivity to whatever insulin is present by adjusting the ratio between fat and lean body mass. Thus, if you currently are taking medications for diabetes, a carefully supervised aerobic exercise program can actually enable you to eliminate oral medications and reduce injected medications.

Fighting Insomnia

Have you ever woken up in the morning feeling refreshed and rejuvenated? So many people don't find this to be the case. They go to bed exhausted and wake up even more exhausted. This phenomenon occurs because their fatigue results from the overtaxing of their adrenal glands through stress. The peaks and dips that often follow a high-sugar diet take a great toll on the body and lead to weariness and exhaustion. I like to call this the "crash-and-burn" cycle. Additionally, during the menopausal years, some women experience insomnia due to hormonal fluctuations.

Aerobic exercise can be an excellent antidote to insomnia, whatever its cause. It helps tire out your body in a healthy way, so that when you crawl between the sheets at night, you are ready for a sound and body-building sleep. Your muscles and bones have been working hard but have been doing so in a health-enhancing fashion.

During perimenopause, when so many women are afflicted by insomnia, exercise is one of the best remedies available. You will notice the difference between your tiredness after a day that included exercise and your tiredness after a day of doing nothing but standing or sitting. And you will certainly feel the difference when you wake up the next morning.

Combating Depression and Stress

Who needs Prozac or Valium when you have exercise? Studies have shown that exercise can be as effective as medication in addressing symptoms of depression and anxiety.

There are several reasons for this. Exercise stimulates the release of endorphins in the brain. These are substances that are responsible for making you feel good. If you're happy, your brain is producing a large quantity of endorphins. Studies have shown that when people behold beauty—a lovely painting or a particularly breathtaking landscape—their brains release endorphins. The same thing happens when they listen to soothing music, pet their favorite cat or horse, or are in the presence of someone they love and trust. If you are sad or depressed, this release of endorphins can help elevate both your energy level and your mood.

Paradoxically, exercise will also help to calm you if you are tense and anxious. Have you ever felt so restless that you need to "just get out" and "burn off" some of the excess energy? After jogging you feel calmer. Sometimes this happens because the exercise actually burns energy-producing sugars that are present in your blood. Exercise also helps to address the extra adrenaline that is produced by your adrenal glands when you are upset. This adrenaline production, often called the "fight-or-flight" response, seems to be a vestige of our ancestors' life in the jungle. When our early ancestors were faced with a physical threat—say, a ferocious animal—their fear caused a burst of adrenaline that enabled them either to fight the threat or flee from it. Nowadays, our "threat" is more likely to be a nasty boss than a charging beast. Yet our bodies still respond with the so-called fight-or-flight response, which causes the heartbeat to quicken, the palms to sweat, and energy levels to rise. Since we cannot physically fight or escape from most of our stressors, the enormous burst of physical energy is wasted and converted into physical anxiety. If the process occurs often enough, we may react by experiencing a variety of stress-related problems.

Exercise controls stress because it gives the body a healthy way to discharge some of that excess energy. The lower heart rate, lower blood pressure, and lower adrenaline levels that are present after exercise provide a direct antidote to the fight-or-flight response and ameliorate some of the physical and emotional symptoms induced by stress.

Boosting Libido

Sexual experience involves a complex set of interactions between your emotions and your hormones. Your partner might have the face of Adonis, the body of Mr. America, and the mind of Albert Einstein, but if your hormones are out of balance, your response to him will be stunted or nonexistent. Exercise can give your sex life a tremendous boost by helping to maintain the inner biochemical environment needed to create and sustain arousal. Restoration of hormonal balance often leads to restoration of sexual arousal.

Exercise boosts libido for another reason: When we feel fit, when our muscles are toned, and when we like the way we look, we generally feel younger and sexier. All of these have a positive impact on the sex drive.

Combating Osteoporosis

Osteoporosis is one of the most serious concerns for women as they travel beyond their menopausal years into older adulthood. In fact, osteoporosis is probably the most common reason why many older women curtail their activities and limit their independence. The brittle bones associated with osteoporosis lead to a slower gait, feelings of weakness, and the risk of hip fracture.

Exercise has been shown to be crucial in the prevention of osteoporosis and even in its reversal. A group of British scientists administered a questionnaire regarding lifestyle to 580 postmenopausal women, age forty-five to sixty-one. They also analyzed the bone mineral density of each participant. The results showed that women who engaged in regular vigorous exercise had greater bone mineral density than those who did not. Many other studies have confirmed this association between exercise and postmenopausal bone health. For example, a Dutch scientific team conducted a rigorous review of the medical literature from 1966 to 1996. They wanted to assess whether most medical studies confirmed the association between osteoporosis prevention or treatment and exercise in postmenopausal women. They concluded that exercise-training programs can, indeed, prevent or reverse bone loss.

Osteoporosis responds best to a combination of aerobic and anaerobic (strength-building) exercises. The word for this combination is *cross-training*. If you engage in an aerobic exercise—such as walking or swimming—and combine it with a strength-building exercise—such as weight lifting—you are building muscle mass and actually increasing the density of your bones. Studies have shown that this type of combined exercise program both prevents and reverses bone loss.

Now that you know *why* you should engage in regular aerobic as well as anaerobic exercise, you're ready to look at how you can do this. We will begin by discussing aerobic exercise—what it is, what it isn't, and how it can be incorporated into your life. Then we will turn our attention to anaerobic, or strength-building, exercises.

Aerobic Exercise

Aerobic exercise, which uses oxygen consistently to burn free-floating and stored body fat as fuel, can be defined as any regular body motion that is sustained for at least twenty minutes at the same pace without stopping. It does not have to be intense or tiring, but it must be regular, steady, and rhythmic.

A few general remarks and caveats are in order before we look at the specific forms of aerobic exercise that you might consider. To begin with, if you have never exercised and are over the age of fifty, then you should definitely get a clean bill of health from your physician before embarking upon a fitness program. Most people can safely initiate a walking program, especially if they start out slowly—by strolling for five minutes, for instance—and work their way up to longer periods of time and a brisker pace. But any other type of exercise—jogging, swimming, bicycling, or dancing, for example—should not be undertaken without the approval of a physician.

Another important warning is to avoid engaging in strenuous outdoor exercise in the heat. During every heat wave, the newspaper bombards us with stories of joggers who become dehydrated and collapse. If you do go outdoors in hot weather, carry a water bottle and use it regularly!

Be sure you do some warm-up stretching exercises before you set out. These will stretch and tone your muscles so that you can more effectively walk, run, swim, bicycle, or whatever you have decided to do. Warm-up exercises are simple. They involve some very gentle stretching to loosen muscles that are stiff from resting, sitting, or standing. They should not be strenuous. You should not contort your body into all sorts of unnatural positions, believing that you are "limbering up." I have patients who have injured themselves in overzealous attempts to engage in stretching exercises.

This brings me to my next point: *Be sensible!* Allow a professional trainer or exercise therapist to give you a warm-up routine, or at least consult a reputable book or video. Videos are available in your local library, bookstore, or video store. They are designed to assist you in any exercise—low impact, medium impact, or high impact—depending on your physical condition. They can even address specific body parts that need work! They will help you to know which movements to avoid and will guide you through your workout from warm-up to cool-down.

Warming up and building up are very important. You should never exercise to the point of exhaustion—let alone beyond it—unless you are in top physical condition. Be realistic about your goals and build up slowly. You will then be sure that your exercise program contributes to your health, rather than detracting from it, and that you have created a regimen that you can sustain over time. You don't have to kill yourself to get into great shape!

Walking

Perhaps the best and most versatile form of aerobic exercise is walking. By this, I don't mean strolling. Nor do I mean the type of slow and irregular walk you might engage in when going up and down supermarket aisles, or window-shopping at the mall. Nor do I mean the short spurt of walking you might do to get from your apartment to the bus stop, or from the office to the cafeteria. For walking to be an effective aerobic exercise, it must challenge the body. In other words, you must find and adopt a pace that is sufficiently brisk to cause your heartbeat to quicken and your body to expend a significant amount of energy. That doesn't mean you must huff and puff. Moreover, to reap the fullest aerobic benefits from your walk, your workout must sustain the same brisk pace.

For this reason walking at a track will probably be more beneficial than walking on the streets near your home. People who come to tracks are usually there to exercise, and you are less likely to get into conversation, become distracted, or be tempted to stop. If you bump into a friend, you can walk together without slowing your pace.

Walking may be the easiest exercise to incorporate into your lifestyle, because you don't need special clothes or special training. You can begin slowly and work up to a brisker pace. If you don't have a track nearby, you can accomplish the same aerobic results by walking in your neighborhood. Perhaps you'll meet some new people, investigate some new areas of your town, or see some pretty flowers you never noticed before. Local walking is fun because it can open your eyes to sights you see each day but may never have really attended to in your haste to get to work or accomplish all your daily tasks. And walking requires no investment of money and minimal investment of time.

As with all exercise, if you're not in shape, you should begin slowly. Start with a five-minute walk, then work up to ten, fifteen, then twenty minutes. You should also increase your speed from a stroll to a brisk and energetic pace. Your goal is to walk at a fast clip for twenty to thirty minutes at a time.

Jogging

In some ways, jogging is a slightly better aerobic exercise than walking, because it presents a greater challenge to the body and therefore burns more calories and builds greater strength in the leg muscles. Joggers report that the emotional benefits of jogging surpass those associated with walking. It's harder to dwell on your problems and sorrows when you are jogging than it is when you are walking. You are more likely to "lose" yourself in your exercise. Moreover, a larger quantity of endorphins is released by your brain, leading to a pleasant after-jog sensation, or even to "runner's high."

Jogging is, however, not free of potential hazards. If sneakers lack sufficient cushioning, the impact of the soles of your feet on hard concrete is jarring to your body and could cause harm to your blood vessels. Jogging is notorious for causing too much stress and strain—particularly on older people who are out of shape and seek to plunge right into a fitness program without building up slowly. Newspapers occasionally carry reports of older people who collapsed while jogging, because the exercise has overtaxed their hearts. Finally, people who raise their legs too high while they jog risk getting "runner's diarrhea"—a condition induced by the excessive massaging of the intestinal walls.

The best way to begin a jogging program is to build up first through walking. After you've succeeded in walking at a brisk pace for, say, half an hour, then you can begin to pick up your pace and lift your knees a little higher. Gradually, you can incorporate five minutes of jogging into your thirty minutes of walking. Then you can cut the walking to twenty minutes and increase the jogging to ten minutes. Continue to do this until you are able to sustain a half-hour jogging session.

If walking isn't sufficiently challenging and jogging is too difficult, you should consider "power walking." Many older adults find that it provides the benefits of challenging, brisk aerobic exercise without some of the problems associated with jogging.

Bicycling

Bicycling is a wonderful form of aerobic exercise. It's fun, it's invigorating, and it's quite versatile. You can bicycle on a flat area, such as a track, or you can bicycle uphill and thereby engage in some focused muscle-strengthening of your thigh and calf muscles.

There are two important pointers for you to consider if you decide to make bicycling your primary form of aerobic exercise.

First, be sure your bicycle is in good shape. You don't need an expensive mountain bike if you're planning to do a half hour on the flat surface of the track, for example, but you will need a bike with gears if you plan to go up and down hills. Your equipment must be appropriate for the type of riding you plan to do.

Second, wear a bicycle helmet! Many cyclists suffer serious head injuries each year because they neglect to take proper precautions to protect their heads in the event of a fall. You're trying to build your health, not destroy it!

Like walking and jogging, bicycling must be taken on gradually. You can't plunge into a full half-hour biking session the first time your feet turn the pedals. Use similar methods to those described for beginning a walking or jogging regimen—begin with a few minutes and gradually work your way up to a sustained half hour. Once you have become accustomed to biking on a smooth surface—say a track designed for cyclists—you can begin negotiating steeper inclines and try your new-found skills all over town.

Swimming

Swimming has great advantages as well as some disadvantages. It is a marvelous aerobic exercise because it involves the whole body, not just the lower extremities. Whether your preferred swimming stroke is the crawl or the backstroke, you are moving your arms, your shoulders, and your head as well as your hips, legs, and feet. You can swim in hot weather without being concerned about becoming dehydrated. If you are asthmatic, swimming is an excellent exercise because it builds lung capacity. You also avoid many airborne allergens—such as pollen, ragweed, and environmental toxins and pollutants—that might affect you if you choose to walk, jog, or ride a bicycle. Swimming is refreshing and can even be exhilarating.

The disadvantage to swimming is that it is not a weight-bearing exercise. The water buoys you up, and although you exert yourself to move through it, you do not actually build muscle mass. So while swimming contributes immensely to cardiovascular health, it does not necessarily contribute to bone density. If osteoporosis is your major concern, you should find a different source of aerobic exercise or be sure to supplement with a weight-training regimen. We will discuss weight-bearing exercises in greater detail on page 138.

Dancing

If you love to dance, you can turn your passion into an aerobic exercise. There are several ways to accomplish this. One is to join a dance class. Dancing of all kinds—disco, square, contra, line, and ballet, for example—all involve some physical activity and are excellent and enjoyable ways to break yourself into regular aerobic exercise. Going to a dance club can also be an invigorating and enjoyable experience.

As you become more committed to your exercise program, you may want to start dancing at home. This will improve your skills. More important, it will create a more rigorous and sustained aerobic activity than you would have on the dance floor of a club, where the songs generally are short, friends come and go, the band takes a break, and people wander over to offer you drinks. A class, also, is not necessarily conducive to the most optimum form of aerobic exercise. The instructor often focuses on specific techniques and steps, so it becomes difficult to sustain a steady twenty-minute dancing session without being rude or disruptive.

My advice is that you do your aerobic dancing at home, and then have a good time on the dance floor or in class, without worrying about whether you're getting enough exercise. When you're dancing at home, select long-playing music, or make your own back-to-back recording of your favorite dance pieces. Be sure the songs are rhythmically similar, because aerobic exercise is effective only if a consistent pace is sustained.

When you dance at home, be sure that you are moving your whole body, and that you are doing so with a consistent set of motions and at a consistent pace. Otherwise, the dancing may be fun but it won't serve as aerobic exercise.

In-Home Aerobic Exercise Equipment

If your responsibilities make it difficult for you to get out of the house, you might consider purchasing a treadmill, indoor trampoline, stair machine, or stationary bicycle. You can set these up in front of the television, if you think that watching TV might help make the exercise more enjoyable and the time pass more quickly. As with outdoor exercise, it is important for you to build up slowly. Stationary bicycles as well as treadmills can be adjusted to less strenuous or more strenuous settings, so that you can gradually work up from an easy pace to one that is more challenging and difficult.

What About Competitive Sports?

Many of you probably enjoy tennis, racquetball, bowling, volleyball, badminton, or table tennis. Competitive sports have great social appeal. Often, friendships are formed or maintained through the regularity of team sports. If you are competitively minded, you might also enjoy the challenge and the thrill of winning. When you leave the tennis court sweaty and triumphant, you feel that you have really exercised.

You're right—you certainly have exercised! But you haven't engaged in the most beneficial and health-building form of aerobic exercise, because the spurts of energy required to run after the ball mean that you're not taking in a sustained and steady supply of oxygen. When you're engaged in the strenuous aspects of the game, your breath comes in fits and starts. Then, after a few minutes, you stop while you tally the score or discuss the set. So by all means, enjoy your tennis or volleyball game. But don't substitute it for consistent aerobic exercise, because it doesn't serve the same purpose in your body.

Setting Up an Aerobic Exercise Program

The most important part of setting up an aerobic exercise program actually takes place before you move a single muscle. You must begin by moving the gray matter in your brain and giving careful thought to which particular form of exercise fits in best with your lifestyle and personal preferences. The mistake that many people make when they begin to exercise is taking on too much too quickly, and in a form that is incompatible with their lifestyle or personality.

If your previous attempts to exercise have left you bored and discouraged, perhaps you will do better if you set up some home exercise equipment in front of the television. You can also obtain some exercise tapes from the library or bookstore, put them into your VCR, and allow yourself to be guided through a complete workout. As mentioned above, a good tape will take you though a session that begins with warm-ups, continues with calisthenics, and concludes with a rhythmic form of exercise.

Exercise tapes can also become boring, though, so you might consider switching among several tapes.

Here's another solution to loneliness and boredom: Join a gym and make some friends while working out. This might take care of the boredom problem as well as provide a supportive environment in which to launch your exercise program.

If you like the outdoors and find yourself tightly scheduled, then walking might be the best exercise for you. Think creatively. Walk, don't drive, to the bus stop—even if you must leave your house a little earlier. Perhaps you can walk from the bus to the office instead of taking the subway. You can also take a shorter lunch break and use twenty minutes of your lunch hour to walk. While you might need to change your shoes, you shouldn't need to change your entire outfit, as you might if you decided to jog or bicycle to work. Walking is the easiest exercise to fit into a workday.

Bicycling is nearly as versatile and convenient as walking. You might have to change your clothes, but you can accomplish errands or even get to work by bicycle—if it's geographically convenient—instead of taking a car, bus, or subway.

If none of these ideas will work for you, then you might simply have to set up a schedule in which you leave the house to go to a gym, swimming pool, or track. There are so many possibilities and options!

The key issue is to establish a regularity of routine. We will discuss how you can do this later in this chapter (page 142).

Let's turn now to strength-building exercises and examine what they are, how they work, and how they should be incorporated into your total exercise program.

Strength-Building Exercises

I've told many clients that I see strength-building exercises as essential to good health, and I've watched them balk and cringe. When I ask them why they react this way, they tell me that they worry about looking like female versions of Charles Atlas, with bulging biceps and monstrous thighs. I always laugh and say that that this isn't what strength training is all about.

So what are strength-building exercises, and what are they meant to accomplish?

Strength-building exercises increase strength by training your muscles to bear increasingly heavier objects, thereby building muscle mass and increasing bone power. Unlike aerobic exercise, strength building is not meant to address issues of circulation, weight loss, or cholesterol. It does not involve the predictable and rhythmic use of oxygen. It focuses on building one particular area of the body, rather than toning up the whole, although the entire body benefits from these exercises, as we discussed earlier in this chapter.

There are many different kinds of strength-building exercises, of which weight lifting is probably the most versatile, portable, and simple. While a gym or a workout facility probably is the most optimal environment for maximizing your exercise possibilities, you can certainly find many helpful exercises that can be performed in the comfort and privacy of your home, with minimal equipment and expense.

If you have never been involved in strength-building exercises, it is crucial that you get a thorough checkup first. These exercises can be very strenuous, and a physician should make sure that you're in sufficiently good shape to undertake them. Even if you're given a completely clean bill of health but you have not exercised for a long time, you should not plunge into a strength-building program without some supervision. Consider going to a reputable gym where you can work out under the guidance of exercise specialists. You can see a physical therapist or a physician who specializes in sports medicine, just to get you started. You can also arrange for a certified fitness trainer to come to your home and work with you a few times to set up regimen that you can then carry out on your own.

If you're in good health and have some experience with exercise, you don't need the same degree of supervision. You can exercise on your own, in a gym, or with the assistance of exercise tapes.

Once again—and most important—be sensible! Educate yourself. Incorrect weight lifting can injure your back. *A Note About Posture* (page 142) will give you some idea of how to engage in safe strength building. If you have any additional questions, be sure to consult a professional.

Now let's have a look at the different types of strength-building exercises and how you can incorporate them into your life.

Types of Weight Lifting

The best way to build muscle mass is through lifting progressively heavier items in a safe and systematic fashion. This isn't done by lifting a heavy laundry basket or heavy suitcases, or by carrying around your five-year-old granddaughter—although a good weight-training program should help you to do all these things with considerably less effort. Building muscle mass through weight lifting is a step-by-step process beginning by lifting very light weights and steadily working your way upward.

You will need two types of weights: those that build the upper body (shoulders, neck, arms, hands, and torso), and those that build the lower body (hips, buttocks, thighs, calves, and feet.) Let's look at each.

Strengthening Your Upper Body   There are three basic types of equipment you can use to strengthen your upper body: hand-held weights, wrist weights, and body bars. Let's look at each one in turn.

Hand-held weights are small versatile weights that are grasped in your hand. If you like to walk, you can hold them in your hand and move your arms to and fro while you walk. You will need to move your arms forward and backward, as well as up and down.

You can also use hand-held weights while exercising in place. Begin by holding the weights in your hands and allowing your hands to dangle at your sides. Slowly bend your elbows, raising the weights, until they are flush to your shoulders. You will look like the letter *w*. Keeping your motions even rather than abrupt, begin to extend your arms over your head until they are straight. Then lower them by reversing the steps you just took.

You will want to do three sets of eight to twelve repetitions. In other words, lift the weights eight times, and then rest for thirty to sixty seconds. Do this again two more times. You may want to start with one set before working up to two or three. As you get stronger, you can increase the number of repetitions to nine, then to ten, and finally to twelve.

When you're first starting out, you should get light weights—say two-pound units. As you get stronger, you can purchase heavier and heavier items. Ideally, your goal is to increase to five to eight pounds per hand. You will probably need to obtain dumbbells, since they are available in heavier weights than hand-held units.

Wrist weights are particularly helpful for walkers, rather than for individuals who wish to do in-place exercises. They are "bracelets" you can attach to your wrists with Velcro or snaps. They have many compartments, each holding a metal peg. You can increase the weight by adding pegs to the compartments, until you have built up to five pounds.

Wrist weights are useful if you wish to walk and need to have your hands free—say if you are on your way to work and you're holding a shopping bag or a book. Because you're not going to be lifting your hands, you won't get the same benefits as you would from hand-held weights, but if this is the only type of weight-bearing exercise you have time for, it is better than nothing.

Body bars are long bars designed to be lifted over your head. You can use them for bicep curls and other exercises, too. They come in different weights, beginning with eight pounds. Ideally, you want to work up to holding a ten- or fifteen-pound bar. Follow the same steps as you would with hand-held weights: Using a light-weight bar, begin with one eight- to twelve-repetition set of each exercise. As you become comfortable, add another set until you have worked your way up to three sets of each exercise. Over the course of time, as the exercise becomes easier and less challenging, you may wish to increase the weight of the bar. You may initially have to decrease the number of repetitions each time you start using a heavier bar.

Strengthening Your Lower Body   Strengthening your lower body—hips, buttocks, leg muscles, and feet—can be accomplished in a number of ways. Again, you accomplish this with aerobic exercise regimens that focus on the use of lower-body muscles. You may begin with a one-pound weight on each ankle and work up to five pounds per ankle when doing a series of lower-body exercises. You can also buy exercise resistance bands that can be used in the comfort of your home, as well as lower body "toning" videotapes that focus on the lower body and buttocks (where most of us need help!). All of these are available at sporting goods stores.

If you have access to a gym, you have many machines to choose from to do weight-bearing exercises with your legs. Gyms also offer classes that focus on the lower and upper body.

A Note About Posture

It is crucial to maintain correct posture when you are lifting weights. If you do not, you might injure yourself. Here are some pointers:

- Make sure your back is straight. It should not be bent forward, or arched.
- Make sure your knees are bent slightly. Do not go into a deep knee bend, but do not keep them rigid.
- Keep your abdominal muscles firm so that they can support your back.

Setting Up a Strength-Building Program

Begin by looking at yourself—your physical health, personal preferences, and lifestyle. These will determine which strength-building exercises you choose, and how you proceed.

If you have time to exercise in place, for example, you might want to purchase home equipment such as a body bar for your upper body or a bench press to strengthen your lower body. Sporting goods stores carry a variety of body-building machines and gyms designed for home use. You might want to set up a workout room right in your house. Equip it with some pretty plants or paintings, a stereo, television, and VCR. Then you can exercise using the guidance of a professional strength-building video-tape or to the background accompaniment of a talk show, movie, or your favorite music.

If you do not have the time to exercise at home or the money to invest in a great deal of home workout equipment, then walking with hand-held or wrist weights should be manageable. These are not expensive and can be incorporated into your existing aerobic exercise regimen without much inconvenience.

As with aerobic exercise, you should begin slowly, with one-pound weights. If you are lifting these in place, then begin with one set of eight repetitions. Gradually work your way up to twelve repetitions. Then, when you are ready, add another set.

As you build your strength, you may want to intensify your program. When exercise stops being a physical challenge and becomes too easy, it loses much of its benefit. You can do this in one of two ways: Either increase the number of repetitions in which you engage or add more weight to the units you are holding. If you are limited in time, the second approach may be more appropriate for you. It will certainly be more appropriate if your weight lifting consists of wearing wrist weights while you walk. There are several excellent brands of wrist weights that can be adjusted to become heavier as you build your strength.

Putting It All Together

It may be overwhelming for you to read about all these different exercises. Perhaps you feel that it's too difficult and complicated to assemble them into a program that you can carry out regularly and effectively.

That's just not so! I have seen dozens of women embark upon life-changing exercise regimens by taking a careful look at their lifestyle and thinking creatively. As I said earlier, you must exercise your brain before you exercise the rest of your body! Get your creative muscles moving and they will guide you in exercising your physical muscles.

Are you a busy business executive? Then walk to work. Instead of carrying a briefcase, use a backpack and free your hands to carry weights. Use wrist weights—it doesn't matter if they look "funny." Your health is more important than the opinions of strangers who might pass you on the street. You've incorporated into a single trip to the office the benefits of aerobic as well as strength-building exercises.

Are you homebound because of caretaking responsibilities? You can set up all the equipment you need right in your living room! While you are watching television, you can use the stationary bicycle, treadmill, or trampoline. After twenty minutes, you can lift weights. If you enjoy music, then turn on your favorite pieces and dance! Music will add rhythm and zest to even the most tedious program.

Don't feel that exercise should be a lonely and isolating process. Consider calling a few friends and starting an exercise group that will rotate from home to home. It will be fun, and you'll have a supportive network of people who will encourage one another to keep up the momentum. Don't give in to the temptation to reward yourselves with ice cream afterward! You can put out some healthy snacks—juice, sliced vegetables and fruits, or whole-grain crackers—to refresh and reward yourselves for a job well done.

Here are a few suggestions to get you started.

Step by Step

If you have led a sedentary lifestyle until now and you feel overwhelmed by the exercise program I've outlined, I'd like to propose a three-level approach that will make exercising more manageable for you.

Level One   Start small, with a short walk once or twice a week after breakfast, lunch, or dinner, or whenever you can fit it in. Even five minutes is better than nothing, because it enables you to establish a new routine and feel a sense of commitment to your program. Of course, if you can start with a longer walk—say, fifteen minutes or so—it would be better.

You can also use an indoor trampoline, step machine, treadmill, or stationary bicycle.

After a month of this new routine, step it up a little. You can do so by adding a few minutes a day and an extra session a week.

Level Two   Some of you may stay at level one for a very long time. Even this small-scale exercise program will be satisfying and will make an enormous difference in your health and well-being. At some point, you may wish to move up to the next level, which is somewhat more comprehensive and rigorous. Here are some suggestions:

- Increase your pace so that you are walking more briskly, or even jogging. This will help you to achieve an even greater fitness level, burn more calories and body fat, and increase your circulation yet further. If you are using exercise equipment, such as a bicycle or treadmill, consider increasing the speed, tension, or upward incline.
- Add some light hand-held weights while you walk or use them while on a stationary bicycle, treadmill, or stepper.
- Increase the amount of time you exercise to thirty minutes.
- Do some light weight-training—say one set—once or twice a week.

Level Three   Level three involves adding more rigorous and intensive exercises to your regimen. When you exercise at this level, you are cross-training. This means that you are combining aerobic and strength-building exercises into a rigorous, unified regimen. Here are a few tips.

- Increase the weight you hold while you engage in aerobic exercises from lighter to heavier wrist or hand-held weights. You can also increase the time you exercise.
- Intensify your weight-training program to include dumbbell curls, overhead presses, or heavier bars.
- Intensify your weight-training program to include more repetitions of each activity and more weight-training sessions each weak. Ideally, you will want to engage in weight lifting two to three times a week.
- Continue to intensify your aerobic exercise by challenging your body further. Increase the speed, tension, or upward incline on your exercise equipment. Increase your pace while walking or running. If you are swimming, consider learning strokes that engage new muscles and body parts.

Some Success Stories

The vignettes below are designed to bring to life some of the exercise suggestions you have just read. Each of you has a unique lifestyle. You have family, friends, employment, responsibilities, and hobbies. Your schedules vary, as do your interests, strengths, and personal commitments. I hope that the three stories below will give you some idea of how you can incorporate exercise into your own unique set of circumstances.

Judy's Story   "I have no time to exercise!" This is probably the most common litany I hear from my patients. I certainly heard this from Judy Q, age fifty-two, who came to see me because she was depressed. Her doctor had recommended Prozac. Judy, nervous about possible side effects, was seeking alternatives.

Judy owns a small flower store about a half-hour drive from her house. The store is open six days a week. Judy must be at the store by 9 A.M. to organize things before the store's official opening at 10. Once the store opens, Judy is on her feet assisting customers until closing time at 6 P.M.

It takes another hour to do all the necessary paperwork connected with the sales of the day. Judy usually arrives home between 7:30 and 8:00 P.M., exhausted. It's all she can do to warm up her food, unwind in front of the television, and collapse into bed.

"No matter how much sleep you get, I'm sure you never feel rested," I told her. "You probably feel tense and anxious, not only depressed."

She stared. "How did you know?"

I smiled. "I'm a scientist, not a psychic. A schedule like yours is rigged to create physical burnout."

Judy and I created an exercise program that she implemented immediately.

She realized that the first half hour of the day was usually downtime. She couldn't remember the last time a customer actually entered the store at 10 A.M. She decided to move a stationary bicycle into the back room of the store and use the half hour between 10:00 and 10:30 to go on the bicycle. "I can prop a book on the handlebars so I won't get bored," she told me. "Maybe then I'll even enjoy exercising!"

"Start slow," I warned her. "Remember that you haven't exercised for many years and you're likely to experience some charley horse."

Judy began by using the bicycle for five minutes, three times a week. After two weeks, she increased to ten minutes and, after a month, she was doing three twenty-minute sessions a week. At the end of two months, she had worked her way up to half an hour. If a customer interrupted her, she made up the time the next day.

After two weeks, Judy began to feel more energetic. After a month, she was waking up every morning refreshed and eager to greet the day. "I can't believe how much better I feel!" she bubbled enthusiastically. She added, "I've attached a reading stand to the bicycle, so I've also gotten some wonderful reading done. I'm working my way through all those books that I always told myself I'd read one day when I had the time. Now I've made the time!"

Judy stepped up her exercise program by adding another exercise session each week and intensifying the tension on her stationary bicycle. Twice a week she began to hold some light weights in her hands. This impeded her reading but enabled her to engage in some weight training while she was doing her aerobic workout. She has sustained this level of exercise and has also retained all the benefits to her physical and emotional health.

Mary's Story "I have osteoporosis and my doctor wants me to start exercising," said sixty-three-year-old Mary W. "But I don't want to."

"Why not?" I asked. "Is it hard for you to find the time?"

"Oh, I have plenty of time on my hands," Mary confessed, looking embarrassed. "In fact, I have nothing but time. I don't have a job. My husband is retired. We spend our days reading, gardening, and baby-sitting for our grandchildren."

"Then what's the problem?" I asked.

"I hate to exercise. It's boring, and I get tired very easily. It seems stupid to make myself pant and sweat if I can just relax in an armchair."

"Exercise doesn't have to be boring or exhausting," I told Mary.

Working with Mary turned out to be easier than I thought. She decided to take her baby grandson out in the stroller every day for a walk, together with her husband. They began with a five-minute stroll and worked up to a half-hour stroll. Once they had built up enough stamina, they began to increase their pace, until they were walking at a fast clip.

I was delighted when Mary, who had worked up to thirty minutes of exercise each day by walking with the stroller, returned for more exercise recommendations. "I feel younger than I did when I was young," she said.

Mary agreed to go to a gym three times a week and work with a trainer on strength-building exercises. I recommended a trainer who was particularly friendly, and Mary found herself looking forward to spending time at the gym. Conversation with the trainer and her fellow exercisers made the time go more quickly, and Mary was never bored.

After several months with the trainer, Mary and her husband went to a hotel with some friends. Mary wore a two-piece bathing suit for the first time in twenty years. She looked so much younger, her friends were convinced that she'd had plastic surgery. Best of all, she began reversing her osteoporosis! Her doctor was amazed when he saw the results of Mary's bone mineral densitometry test a year after she started her exercise program. He called his secretary to make sure Mary's test results hadn't been confused with someone else's. "I can't believe it. Your bone mineral density has improved! I've never seen anything like this before."

Nan's Story Nan A, a forty-eight-year-old lawyer, was experiencing debilitating hot flashes. "The last one happened in court, right in front of the judge, as I approached the bench," she said. "I was nervous about the case, and I found myself stammering and feeling awful. My gynecologist suggested HRT, but there's a history of breast cancer in my family. I don't want to take the risk."

I outlined the total menopause program, and she nodded briskly, taking notes on diet and supplements. When I got to exercise, she smiled and closed her notebook. "I play tennis twice a week. I don't need more exercise."

"Tennis is a good beginning, but I think you need to do more than that."

"I don't want to give up my tennis nights," Nan protested. "They're very important to me. And there's no other time to exercise. I see clients all day."

As we examined Nan's schedule, we realized that she could walk from the bus station to work, instead of taking a taxi. This would give her a solid twenty-minute stretch of time twice a day. She felt she could incorporate two fifteen-minute slots of time each week to do some weight lifting.

The plan was very effective. Nancy began to feel a reduction in hot flashes, as well as a general sense of greater well-being. "Best of all," she reported enthusiastically a few months later, "my tennis is much better. I'm more alert and coordinated, and I have a lot more stamina."

You Can Do It, Too

The stories of Judy, Mary, and Nan all illustrate how—with a little creativity and commitment—exercise can be smoothly incorporated into your lifestyle, no matter how crazy, hectic, or tightly scheduled your time may be. Exercise also does not have to be dull and dreary. In the right environment, it can be stimulating and enjoyable, and provide fun that will rebound positively in all the other areas of your life.

Six

Attitude and Emotions
During Menopause

In chapter 1, we took a quick glance at some of the attitudes that Western women bring to their experience of perimenopause and menopause. We mentioned that all too many American women view this natural process with dread. This chapter will take a more careful look at the beliefs of American women about aging in general, and menopause in particular, focusing on the basis of those beliefs, and on how those beliefs are changing. We will then look at specific perimenopausal and postmenopausal emotional difficulties, and suggest an array of techniques you can use to address them.

Western Attitudes Toward Women's Aging

If you visit Japan, you will notice a fascinating phenomenon. Age is associated with superior wisdom, and older women are regarded with veneration. They are considered to be the family matriarchs whose opinion is valued and whose guidance is sought. If you travel through Africa or Aboriginal Australia, you will encounter a similar phenomenon.

Not so in the United States! You have only to turn on your television to be bombarded by products designed to promote youth and delay or negate aging. In our twenty-something-oriented society, older people are progressively squeezed out of the workforce and then marginalized. Seniors are regarded as being out of touch with today's state-of-the-art technology, and therefore out of touch with society as a whole. This is terribly sad and unfortunate, because older people have a great deal of wisdom and life experience to offer younger people. As the population ages and medical science continues to develop new means of prolonging life, we will see larger numbers of Americans joining the "senior citizen" ranks, and it will become even more important for younger individuals to realize how much older people have to offer.

As hard as it is to feel marginalized by a society to which you once belonged, I believe that the central reason people regard aging with dread is physical rather than social. Aging is associated with illness, loss of physical or mental faculties, and diminished sexual attractiveness or desire. But none of these feared phenomena has to happen! A healthy lifestyle and a positive attitude can keep people young in body and spirit, even while they are aging chronologically.

It seems as though women approaching menopause are beginning to reexamine their attitudes toward aging. A 1998 study conducted by the Gallup Organization revealed that American women are taking a more positive attitude toward aging. The organization interviewed a nationally random sample of 752 American women, age fifty to sixty-five, who had had their last menstrual period at least one year prior to the interview. More than half reported that they are "happier and more fulfilled" than they were in their twenties, thirties, or forties. They reported improvement in family life, sense of personal fulfillment, ability to focus on hobbies, and relationships. Approximately three quarters reported that they feel themselves to be better educated than their mothers and grandmothers, and that they used the knowledge available to them to make some kind of lifestyle change at the beginning of menopause or middle age. These changes included alteration of nutritional habits, exercise, stress reduction, reduction in alcohol or nicotine consumption, and exploration of conventional or alternative approaches to hormone replacement.

This is a very encouraging study. If these participants are representative of the population as a whole, then women are beginning to take a different attitude toward aging and are starting to realize that life gets better as menopause approaches, and even better afterward.

Sadly, I don't think that this is a sufficiently representative sample. Most of my patients, and most of the women I meet on lecture tours and in my other travels, express fear of menopause and its supposed ravages.

I'd like to briefly address the most oft-stated fears, before turning my attention to the more realistic concerns of the emotional roller coaster that so many women experience during the perimenopausal and post-menopausal years.

Why Are We All So Scared?

In listening to women talk about their fears, four emerge as central. Women are afraid of losing their sexual attractiveness. They are afraid of losing their ability to feel sexual. They are worried about physical decline, and they are afraid that they will be put on the shelf by our youth-worshiping society. Let's look at each of these in turn.

Fear of Losing Sexual Attractiveness

Do you peer anxiously into the mirror, straining to see if a new wrinkle has started etching its way into your face? Do you dye your hair, fearing that gray or white will make you look too old? If so, you are not alone. The media and our culture promote the notion that only a "young-looking" woman is beautiful.

It may surprise you to learn that American men—especially those in your age group—do not necessarily regard younger women as more beautiful than older women. Many middle-aged men value the physical appearance of women their own age, rather than that of considerably younger women. The determinants of attractiveness seem to have less to do with hair color and wrinkles and more to do with general vitality, vibrancy, health, and animation. Maturity is not a liability. It's an asset.

My opinion, based on my research as well as my clinical experience, is that women with a good self-image and positive energy—no matter how old they are—attract men. The men they attract tend to be healthy, well-balanced individuals who appreciate these values and qualities in the women they date. So if you are single and interested in becoming involved with a man, take heart. Blooming health and love of life are the best formulas for attracting men with sound judgment and values—men who will appreciate you.

If you are married or already involved in a relationship, you have some wonderful years to look forward to. A whole new chapter of your life is beginning—one that can proceed unencumbered by young children and the stresses that probably marked the early years of your marriage. I'll address this more fully in "Improving Your Relationship," on page 161.

Fear of Losing Sexual Desire

Some of my patients have expressed anxiety that, as they age, they will lose interest in sex. When I question them further, I realize that this fear is based on a network of misunderstandings that mesh to form the notion that postmenopausal women are some kind of sexless species, and that passion is reserved for teenagers. These misunderstandings include the belief that the hormonal changes that accompany menopause rob women of the biochemical "juices" necessary to make them aroused or orgasmic; that vaginal dryness is inevitable and renders sex painful; that older people "just don't want it" anymore; and that sex in older people is somehow embarrassing and inappropriate.

Biochemical changes may or may not weaken your libido, and if they do, this book is filled with strategies that will help you restore it. We discussed diet and exercise in chapters 3 and 5, respectively, and how each could have a positive impact on libido. Chapter 4 taught you about supplements you can take if your relationship is otherwise good but you find your sexuality waning. And chapter 7 will focus on safe hormone replacement, and how androgen supplementation can restore possibly diminished sexual desire. *Hormones will fluctuate during this time of your life, but your sexual desire not only can remain intact but can actually grow!*

It is also important to remember that sexual feelings are as much mental as physical. Belief in your unattractiveness or unsexiness will attack your libido as surely as changes in estrogen or androgen levels. Your sexuality has a far better chance of remaining healthy and strong if you continue to see yourself as a sexual being. To that end, pamper yourself a little bit, possibly—if you are like so many other women—for the first time in your life. Take a long bubble bath, and relish the feeling of sensuality and relaxation it gives your body. (Now just think back: Did you ever soak in the tub when the kids were small or when you were struggling over term papers in college?) Buy yourself pretty undergarments and nightgowns. Purchase clothes and makeup that help you feel good about yourself. Look in the mirror and smile at the face that greets you, remembering that it is the face of a beautiful woman.

Fear of Physical Decline

Perhaps the most common source of anxiety is the fear that rapid aging and physical decline lie in store after menopause. Women often express concern about losing their hearing, vision, strength, and mental acuity. They worry about heart disease, stroke, and cancer. For some reason, the two most common fears of aging concern "senility" (Alzheimer's disease) and hearing loss. Too many women anticipate a future spent as a shuffling old lady mumbling gibberish to herself, except when she's cupping her ear and shouting, "What's that you just said?"

This is an absolutely unnecessary—and indeed, wholly improbable— scenario. I'm going to shock you by saying that with good nutrition, proper exercise, a positive attitude, and appropriate use of nutritional supplements, you can be healthier in mind and body during the second half of your life than you were during the first! The measures we've been discussing throughout this book will give your body the best opportunity to rid itself of toxins, strengthen the immune system, build cardiovascular health, and sharpen your mental acuity.

Fear of Becoming Less Valued by Society

So many of my patients have worried about being pushed to the edges of a society that places its greatest premium on youth. They point out that in the job market, promotions and new jobs almost inevitably are given to younger people, and that they are often edged in not-so-subtle ways toward retirement.

Here's what I say: Take the retirement and use it for personal growth and to build relationships! If your company is foolish enough to overlook your gifts and the formidable contributions you can make, then accept retirement joyously and begin to build your life in new and creative directions. Look at all the things you have always wanted to do. Perhaps you've dreamed of traveling. Perhaps you've wanted to devote more time to your hobbies. Retirement gives you the chance to embrace the dreams you've never been able to fulfill and perhaps even turn them into new careers if you feel that you need—for financial or personal reasons—to continue being part of the workforce.

Do you love to garden? There is an array of creative ways you can turn that passion into a hobby or a source of income. Do you love to sew? Play the piano? Bake? Read books? Draw? Have you always wanted to work with young children, sick people, or animals? You can deepen your involvement in any of these areas, either as hobbies or as new careers. There are also organizations in which retired people can volunteer their expertise to help younger people build their own careers.

You may wish to go back to school to take the classes you never had time to attend when you were young. Most communities have adult-education centers, and most colleges have continuing-education programs. Your coursework can be oriented either toward personal growth and education or toward a degree that will equip you to embark upon a new career of some sort. You can also meet like-minded people and develop a new social network. My experience is that when older adults go back to school, they wind up being straight-A students!

I think that these are the most exciting years of your life, because so many options and opportunities are available to people of all ages. As America's older population continues to grow and older people claim the respect that is rightfully theirs, I believe that social attitudes will change as well.

Addressing Your Emotions

As we've seen, the perimenopausal and postmenopausal years can be a time of enormous personal growth. You can be a happier and healthier person than you ever were.

I'm not denying, however, that this is an emotionally challenging time. Most human beings tend to resist change. This psychological phenomenon has its roots in a physiological phenomenon, well noted and established by scientists. The body is continually seeking *homeostasis*. It tries to avoid change. This is, for example, why it is often so hard to lose weight. You are working *against* your body's desire to remain the same.

The emotional selves, too, seem to prefer sameness, and most of us find change to be frightening. Moreover, the reality is that during menopause, our hormones are going through changes. These *can* affect your mood. In addition to the nutritional, hormonal, and exercise-based approaches discussed elsewhere in this book, there are several psychological approaches and techniques that will help you get through this transition and emerge stronger and happier than you were before.

Relaxation Techniques

If you find yourself tense or anxious during this time in your life, you can try a few simple techniques for altering your state of mind. Numerous studies have shown that anxiety responds well to mind-body techniques designed to induce a state of deep relaxation. The heartbeat slows down, respiration assumes a deep and steady rhythm, and tight muscles begin to loosen up. Relaxation techniques—like exercise regimens—should be integrated into your life based on your lifestyle and needs. Some of the most common and helpful tools are biofeedback, prayer, and meditation.

Biofeedback   Biofeedback is a technique with many far-reaching applications. It has been used effectively in pain reduction, retraining of pelvic floor muscles to address urinary incontinence, and building attention span in children with learning disabilities or Attention Deficit Disorder—to name just a few. It is particularly helpful in teaching people of all ages and in all situations how to relax.

We generally think of our brain waves, heartbeat, and respiration as being out of our control. They are part of our *autonomic nervous system* and do not, as a rule, respond to our conscious commands. Biofeedback helps to bridge the gap, as it were, between our conscious intention and our physical functions. It teaches us to consciously regulate bodily functions that are usually unconscious.

When we are relaxed, our brain waves are actually different from the ones produced when we are tense, or when we are in a creative mode, or when we are asleep. Our brains produce alpha, beta, gamma, and theta waves. Alpha waves are responsible for inducing a state of relaxation in us. We can teach our brains to operate in the alpha mode through biofeedback.

During a biofeedback session, sensors attached to your head record what is happening in your body, and a monitor or screen projects an image that shows the type of brain waves being produced. This image is the "feedback" that guides you in increasing the alpha waves associated with relaxation. While biofeedback is generally done in an office environment with a trained specialist, you can obtain small, hand-held monitors to enable you to do biofeedback in your own home.

Once you have learned to induce a state of deep relaxation using a machine, you can begin to transfer that skill into areas outside the office of the biofeedback practitioner. If you find yourself in a difficult confrontation at work, in a traffic jam, or in an unpleasant scene with your partner or children, you know that you have the ability to relax yourself by using skills you've developed during biofeedback training. Once you're relaxed, you will have more clarity to handle your situation effectively, creatively, and with minimum stress.

Prayer   Scientists recently have begun to study the effects of prayer on the individual praying. Numerous studies have pointed to the positive effects that prayer has on heartbeat, respiration, and relaxation levels. I am not a theologian and do not take a stance on the metaphysical meaning of these studies. I am a scientist and can say with confidence that if these studies were supporting the salutory effect of some herb on anxiety levels and there were no negative side effects or risks associated with that herb, I would wholeheartedly recommend it.

Prayer is a very personal activity, and how you pray will emanate from your worldview and religious orientation. I encourage you to explore your beliefs about prayer and explore the possibility of expanding your definition and understanding of this ancient and comforting activity. You will find a helpful reading list in the "Suggestions for Further Reading" section of this book (p. 193).

One of the reasons people find prayer to be helpful is that they are connecting with a force greater than themselves. Studies have shown that individuals with a spiritual orientation of some sort usually withstand adverse circumstances more successfully than others. Prayer usually reflects a spiritual worldview that can help you through life's changes, including the "change of life."

Meditation   Do you associate meditation with drugged-out sixties hippies or flaky New Age types? If so, you're missing the point of what meditation is and how powerful it can be as a health-promoting tool.

Like biofeedback, meditation can bring about relaxation on the deepest level, flooding the brain with alpha waves and regulating and slowing heartbeat and respiration. An increasing number of scientists are studying the positive effects that meditation has on all aspects of health—physical as well as mental.

While meditation may have its roots in Eastern religions, it has become thoroughly Westernized. For example, Harvard cardiologist Herbert Benson, M.D., adapted transcendental meditation (TM)—which originated in the Hindu tradition—to the needs of his American patients by secularizing many of its religious components. Other scientists have followed suit, and a wealth of information and techniques is now available.

Simply put, meditation is a process that generates a deep state of relaxation in a relatively short period of time. It enables you to still your mind of all its customary anxiety-induced chatter by finding a relaxing position (usually cross-legged or in a straight-backed chair) and focusing on a single object (such as a picture, flower, or holy object) or sound. In TM, for example, the meditator is assigned a special word, called a *mantra,* by a spiritual teacher and is told to repeat and concentrate on that word. Dr. Benson suggests that people can select any word or syllable that is meaningful to them. The changes in brain waves will be the same. Other meditational practices involve making your breath the focus of your concentration, or counting slowly from one to ten repeatedly.

What's nice about meditation is that you don't need electronic equipment or the help of a practitioner. You can meditate in your home, your office, your car, or your garden. Meditation is versatile and highly adaptable to your lifestyle. If you are a "morning person," you can wake up twenty minutes earlier and meditate before work. If you are a night owl, you can meditate at night when the house quiets down. If you have a private office at work, you can close the door during lunch hour. And although meditation is most effective if performed for at least twenty minutes at a sitting, taking a short meditation break of a few minutes at work might serve as a "reset button" if you are tense, or if you'd simply like to clear your mind.

I can hear you saying, "But I don't have time for meditation!" Here, too, you will have to be creative. If you have a busy household, you will have to inform your family members that you need this time to yourself and they shouldn't disturb you. (It's time for them to learn to honor your needs, if they haven't already done so!) You may need to leave the house earlier, or take a sandwich to work so that lunch takes less time and you have some leftover minutes for meditation. Use your ingenuity, and you'll find out meditation actually helps you think more creatively and with greater clarity.

The reading list provided in the "Suggestions for Further Reading" section of this book will help you to get started on a meditational program that conforms to your personal ideology, and also fits your lifestyle.

Exercise-Based Meditation There are several powerful techniques that join meditation with a series of bodily motions. Tai chi, qi gong, and yoga are systems that combine a series of slow physical motions designed to align, stretch, and tone various body parts with meditation. If you are a person who prefers physical activity to sitting, one of these approaches may be appropriate for you.

Tai Chi and Qi Gong Tai chi and qi gong both originate in China. While they have very different origins, they share the same set of philosophical assumptions and premises. Both schools teach that the mind, body, and spirit are linked, and that good health involves a balance among all these three aspects of the human being. Both schools teach that health is also contingent upon balance in the *qi,* the vital life force, or energy, that circulates through the body. The body motions and postures taught by practitioners of tai chi and qi gong are designed to redirect and balance misaligned energy flow.

The full name of tai chi is actually *tai chi chuan*—Chinese for supreme ultimate fist. Tai chi, sometimes referred to as shadow boxing, originated in China in the thirteenth century, although the martial arts principles on which it is based are much older. The first references to it are found in seventeenth-century Chinese literature. Qi gong—which is Chinese for the art of cultivating internal energy—is far more ancient, dating back over two thousand years.

Tai chi and qi gong both involve performing a series of gently executed postures, with intense concentration. The positions are believed to stimulate and redirect the flow of *qi* and to facilitate heightened concentration and relaxation.

Yoga Like tai chi and qi gong, yoga is an ancient movement-based meditational practice. Its origins in India date back several thousand years, and its philosophical underpinnings lie in Hindu religious teachings.

Yoga involves a series of postures designed to realign or strengthen various body parts and also to create a state of intense concentration and calm. Yoga is a useful physical exercise and a wonderful source of relaxation.

Counseling

Any time of transition involves some challenges and difficulties. These are often exacerbated by unresolved issues from earlier times in your life. For example, childhood issues of physical, sexual, or emotional abuse that have not been adequately addressed may resurface during peri- and postmenopause. So, too, may traumatic experiences that occurred during your adult years. By "trauma" I don't mean only the ostensible and obviously traumatic events, such as illness experienced by yourself or a family member, death of a loved one, a sexual or physical assault, or a serious accident. Job loss, divorce, estrangement from a family member, or a move to a new area can be equally traumatic. Indeed, any event that triggers intense emotional pain can be correctly classified as a trauma.

My clinical experience has shown me that people who are still suffering from unresolved painful emotions will have a more difficult menopause. They will experience more savage hot flashes and more brutal mood swings and will have a generally harder time. Again and again I hear patients who have come to see me because of physical symptoms such as headaches begin to talk about their father who beat them, or their mother who never paid attention to them. I urge them to get into some therapeutic program that will enable them to lay their childhood demons to rest and move on with their lives. I tell that that they should see menopause as a gift and an opportunity to put these painful issues behind them once and for all.

There are several different types of counseling settings that I recommend to my patients, depending on their needs. Some patients have found a combination of all three to be helpful.

Individual Counseling   If you are experiencing a midlife crisis, remembering a childhood or other trauma, or going through depression, my advice would be for you to start by setting up an appointment to see a therapist on a one-on-one basis. There are many different types of mental health professionals who might be helpful to you, including psychiatrists, psychologists, social workers, licensed mental health counselors, and members of the clergy. You can locate these individuals through local referral services, your primary care physician, mental health centers or religious institutions, or through friends who might have sought counseling themselves.

You may have to interview several people before you find someone with whom you really "click." The practitioner's degree—M.S.W., Ph.D., Psy.D.—matters less than the feeling you get from the person. Are you comfortable with him or her? Do you feel that this therapist understands you and your situation? Can you open up and express yourself freely? Is this individual committed to helping you grow?

If you are dealing with specific issues such as sexual abuse or addiction, you may need to find a counselor who specializes in treating people who are struggling with these issues.

Seeking therapy doesn't mean you are crazy or mentally imbalanced. Therapy is for healthy individuals who want to become healthier, happier, and whole. Nor do you have to be in therapy for years. Most mental health practitioners are moving away from the tenets of Freudian analysis, with its protracted treatment plans. They prefer short-term insight therapy and highly focused interventions. A good therapist will not keep you in treatment for years, unless you are struggling with a complex or deeply entrenched trauma, or set of traumas, that require some time to heal.

Group Settings   A group can create a powerful healing environment. People who are struggling with the same issues and circumstances as you are can give you perspective and moral support. There are many women's groups. Some meet to talk about specific issues—family, illness, aging, employment, divorce, or caring for an elderly or infirm parent. Others are more general and provide a comfortable and supportive forum in which to make new friends and air general concerns. You can locate a support group through your own therapist, through a local mental health center, or through local community centers.

As a clinician who works with many patients, I have discovered that an alarming number of people have been affected by addiction—their own or that of a close family member. So many of my patients recount stories of sad childhoods due to the alcoholism of a parent. Some are still struggling with the repercussions that their painful childhood circumstances have had on their adult relationships with family and friends. If you are dealing with issues surrounding addiction, I would urge you to attend a group such as Alcoholics Anonymous or Al-Anon, or any other twelve-step program that specializes in the particular issue you're confronting.

There are many excellent organizations that arrange group experiences, such as retreats, regular and ongoing support or self-help groups, and intensive seminars. The Option Process and Silva Mind Control are two examples. You will find additional suggestions in Resources (page 195).

Marital Counseling   In the section below, called "Improving Your Relationship," we will look at some simple and effective ways to enhance your relationship with your husband or partner. But it may be that these are not sufficient to address issues that are arising between you. Times of stress or transition can heighten unresolved marital issues. Your needs may change and you may have less tolerance, for example, for your partner's workaholism and his long hours at the office. If you have experienced sexual problems during the marriage, these may intensify as you—and he—go through the physical changes associated with midlife and aging.

It is important for you to get help now, so that you can maximize the time you both have together. Life is too precious to waste on unsatisfying relationships. A marriage counselor can help you resolve these difficulties by bringing them out into the open, assisting you in communicating with each other, teaching problem-solving techniques, identifying negative patterns that you may have to work on in individual counseling, and facilitating new ways of interacting with each other. Working out the kinks in your marriage so that you feel renewed love, closeness, and companionship can make the years that lie ahead of you even better than the years that lie behind you.

Improving Your Relationship

All marriages go through changes as each member of the couple grows and evolves, and as life circumstances shift. Times of stress and transition—the birth of a new baby, a move to a new home, job loss or the taking on of a new job, illness of family members—all place strain on a couple.

Perimenopause and menopause challenge a relationship because they involve physical as well as emotional changes. It is particularly important to nurture your relationship at this time. Here are a few suggestions.

Communicate with Your Partner   It's amazing how many difficulties can be resolved if you take this simple piece of advice. If you are worried about your attractiveness, if you feel tired or moody, or if your body feels as though it suddenly does not belong to you, sharing your feelings with your partner will help him to understand what you are going through. He will probably be much more understanding of your needs if you express how you're feeling and explain exactly how you want him to support you.

It is important to emphasize that your partner doesn't have to "solve" anything. Some studies suggest that men and women approach problems differently. Women are more likely to share their concerns just to "vent," and appreciate someone who can listen and empathize. Men are more likely to share their concerns as a problem-solving technique and to clam up if they feel there's no solution available. Conversely, women are more likely to *offer* support, empathy, and a listening ear to someone else's problem, while men are more likely to want to offer solutions and become frustrated if that isn't possible.

So when you talk about your problems, make clear to your partner when and how he can be helpful. ("It would help if we could just cuddle for a while . . ." "When I'm tired, I want someone else to do the cooking . . .") If there are no concrete steps he can take, tell him that you are looking for his friendship, support, and listening ear.

It's also important to encourage your partner to communicate his concerns to you. He may have his own misconceptions and assumptions about menopause and aging, and it is important for you to hear them and deal with any issues that might arise for him.

Understand That Men Age, Too   While you are going through your midlife transition, your husband or partner is going through his. He, too, may be experiencing hormonal fluctuations. He may be experiencing prostate problems that affect both his urinary and his sexual functioning. Additionally, he may be worried about his own sexual attractiveness and desirability, about his career and future in the youth-oriented marketplace, and about aging.

This is the time to educate yourself about what's going on in his body and, more important, what's going on in his mind and heart. Communication is essential. Offer as much support and encouragement as you can, and be sure to tell him regularly how much you love him, and how sexy you still think he is.

Take Time Together   A wonderful way to help your relationship not only weather the transition but also grow and thrive is to take extra time to enjoy special activities together. Now that the children have grown up and you have freedoms you never had perhaps in all your married life, you can travel together. If work, finances, or other commitments don't allow for world travel, you can still take day or weekend trips. Make time to go to movies or concerts, take walks in the park, or get involved in an activity you both love, like bowling, bridge, cooking, or language classes. Take extra time to just *be* together—cuddle, make love, be romantic, and try new activities.

Of course, don't forget the old routines that have brought you pleasure and comfort until now. It's important not to rush to overturn your established lives. Enjoy what you've always enjoyed, but take extra time to create new areas of sharing as well.

Reaching Out for Support

American women often are very isolated. Whether we live in a crowded apartment building in a big city or in a house on a tree-lined suburban street, many us of barely know our neighbors. For the most part, we do not live in the close-knit communities that characterize small towns or villages in other countries.

Life changes and transitions can be very difficult if you are going through them alone. If you do not have a circle of supportive friends— preferably women who are going through a similar phase of their lives— then create one. Don't be shy about striking up conversations with women you meet at the track or in the library. Chances are that they'll be as appreciative of your friendship as you'll be of theirs.

If you already have some friends, consider creating an informal support group to share common issues and concerns. You'll be amazed how much companionship there will be, and how much better you can feel!

Becoming Venerable

You will discover that as you implement these suggestions and become the thriving, vibrant, powerful woman you were meant to be, people will seek out your company. Your family will ask you for advice, and people of all ages will value your input. Far from being marginalized, you will be centralized by the people who know you.

Seven

HRT Revisited—Safely

Some of my patients, perhaps responding to the urging of physicians who strongly advocate conventional HRT, feel that they want to try some kind of hormone replacement. They believe that diet and nutritional supplements are not sufficient to provide them with vitality and comfort as they travel the menopausal highway. Many are particularly concerned that alternative approaches will not protect them against the ravages of cardiovascular disease and osteoporosis.

If you also feel uneasy about approaching perimenopause and postmenopause without hormonal therapy, I will tell you what I tell these concerned patients. I believe that diet, exercise, and nutritional supplements are enough to provide you with a solid, sound, and reliable HRT alternative. But if you disagree, there are some safe hormone therapies available. Here's the most important caveat: Don't use them as a substitute for responsible living! A healthy diet and a balanced exercise program are essential, whether or not you're using hormone replacement therapy. In fact, the more balanced your diet, and the more you are addressing your menopausal needs with nutritional supplements and vitamins, the less hormone replacement you are likely to need. Hormones can be added to your holistic health program—but with caution and prudence. This chapter will teach you how to do that. You will learn how to find out whether you actually do have a hormonal deficiency, which particular hormones must be replaced, in which quantities, and at which times of the month.

This chapter is different from the other chapters in this book because you cannot use it on your own. Putting into practice the ideas outlined below requires the cooperation, participation, and guidance of your physician. Sadly, some physicians may not even be familiar with this approach to HRT! It is my hope that this chapter will provide you with enough information to be an educated consumer so that you can approach your physician with a sound and responsible approach to hormone replacement. An honest, compassionate, and open-minded physician will help you to apply what you have learned and create a hormonal regimen that is tailor-made for your biochemical profile. The Resources section (page 195) will suggest some organizations that can help you find a doctor.

Which Hormones Does My Body Produce?

Your body produces many hormones throughout your lifetime. Hormones are substances produced in one part of the body that travel through the blood to produce a reaction in another part of the body. This chapter focuses specifically on what are called sex steroid hormones. These are hormones intimately connected with your reproductive cycle, although some perform other functions in the body as well. As you know from chapter 2, there are five major hormones that are affected by menopause: estrogen, progesterone, testosterone, cortisol, and DHEA.

We briefly discussed some of the functions of these hormones earlier in the book. Table 7:1 provides greater detail about what each of these important substances does in your body.

Table 7:1

Name of Hormone	Major Functions
Estrogen	• Promotes sexual maturation. • Promotes fertility through stimulating ovulation. • Responsible for the first phase of the menstrual cycle. • Responsible for lactation.

	• Promotes cardiovascular health. • Promotes skin elasticity. • Contributes to bone density, preventing osteoporosis. • Contributes to the elasticity of the urinary tract, preventing incontinence. • Contributes to the moisture and suppleness of the vaginal tract, preventing vaginal atrophy. • Relieves hot flashes.
Progesterone	• Modulates estrogen levels. • Relieves some menopausal discomforts, such as hot flashes. • Responsible for the second phase of the menstrual cycle. • Necessary for fertility and maintaining pregnancy. • Enhances mood. • Has a calming effect. • Regulates fluid balance. • Decreases risk of endometrial cancer.
Testosterone	• Builds and maintains muscle mass. • Builds and maintains bone density, preventing and/or treating osteoporosis. • Maintains healthy ligaments. • Increases energy, libido, and assertiveness. • Enhances immune functions.
DHEA	• Contributes to the body's ability to manufacture estrogen, progesterone, and testosterone. • Enhances brain functions such as memory, alertness, and concentration. • Enhances immune function. • Builds and maintains muscle mass.

	• Builds and maintains bone density. • Maintains healthy ligaments. • Contributes to libido. • May protect against Alzheimer's disease. • May protect against cardiovascular disease. • Protects against the effects of stress.
Cortisol	• Modulates response to stress, trauma, and crisis. • Increases energy. • Assists in the metabolism and utilization of fats, protein, and carbohydrates. • Helps regulate blood pressure. • Enhances the integrity of blood vessels. • Modulates pain. • Reduces allergic and inflammatory response.

Why Should My Hormone Levels Be Assessed?

Now that you are familiar with the names and functions of the sex steroid hormones, the question is whether each of these hormones is being produced in your body in the correct amount so that it can do the job it is supposed to do. Are your levels too high? Too low? Entirely normal?

This question may come as a surprise to your doctor, who might assume that your hormonal levels are low if you are experiencing a series of symptoms, such as hot flashes or fatigue. At that point, he or she might put you on a course of HRT treatments. If your physician is like many others, the course of treatment will be one of two or three standard regimens routinely prescribed for patients with your symptoms. Why? Because standard HRT usually is not individualized. This means that HRT often does not address the actual problem. A 1999 survey conducted by the American Association of Clinical Endocrinologists, for example, pointed out that most women are routinely placed on HRT before other causes of their symptoms—causes such as thyroid malfunction—are properly investigated. This survey led the National Thyroid Association to launch a campaign called "Thyroid: the Missing *T* in HRT." I cannot emphasize enough how many women remain symptomatic even after a course of HRT. Many of these women eventually undergo hormone testing only to discover that their estrogen levels are actually too high, while their progesterone or testosterone levels are abysmally low! Give them a few milligrams of testosterone, and their hot flashes disappear, their libido returns, and they feel healthy and rejuvenated.

Clearly, if you want to embark upon a responsible course of hormonal therapy, you must find the true cause of any symptoms you are experiencing. To begin with, of course, your physician must determine if the problem actually is hormonal, or if it has another cause. If, in fact, the problem is hormone based, it is vital to get an accurate hormonal profile so that you will know precisely which hormones need adjustment. The next section will examine the best way in which your physician can make this important determination.

How Should My Hormone Levels Be Assessed?

In order to understand the most effective way of assessing your hormonal levels, it is necessary to understand the different kinds of hormones and how each one is measured.

When your hormones are released into your bloodstream, most of them bind to protein. These *bound hormones* may be circulating in your system but are inactive. They cannot bind with receptors and create a response. The small percentage (about 1 to 10 percent) of free hormones remain unattached, or *bioavailable*. These are available to bind with your receptors and bring about immediate responses in your body.

Assessing your total hormonal levels is less useful than assessing your free hormonal levels. Why? Because the bound hormones are not the ones that are going to work to counterbalance hot flashes, for example, or to provide extra energy and libido. The free hormones are responsible for these and other functions, so it is the free hormones that must be measured.

Is Your Mouth Watering?

If you're looking for a physician to guide you through a hormonal program, you should start by finding someone who is well versed in a new and wonderful method of hormone testing—the saliva test.

Actually, the salivary hormone test isn't really "new." It's been around for a while but has been used primarily for research purposes and to assess whether a pregnant woman is at risk for preterm labor. Only recently has it become available for patients wishing to create a hormonal program shaped to their needs.

Why Is the Saliva Test More Accurate Than a Blood Test?

Because they are not bound to proteins in the bloodstream, are not yet attached to hormone receptors, and are therefore bioavailable, free hormones find their way into your saliva. They enter through cells in your salivary glands. Measuring salivary hormone levels provides an excellent and highly accurate way to assess the amount of free hormones available to interact with your hormone receptors.

Salivary tests are far more accurate than blood tests because blood tests only measure the *total* rather than the *free* estradiol levels in the blood. To be sure, a good mathematician might take the total estradiol level, whip out a calculator, and estimate the amount of free estradiol through a simple calculation. But the patient is nevertheless receiving an approximation rather than an exact figure. This may not sound serious, but it actually is. Responsible medicine is predicated on accuracy of dosages. The apparently minuscule difference between one and two milligrams, for example, is essential if you are rectifying a biochemical imbalance in the body—which is exactly what you are trying to do through HRT. The saliva test measures free hormonal levels quite accurately.

There is a highly practical additional factor that renders saliva tests more accurate and useful than blood tests. Most physicians prescribe hormonal blood tests on a one-shot-deal basis. Your vein is punctured once, and you get your "read-outs" a few days later. You are generally not told to come at any particular time of day, and you show up only once.

In actuality, the time of day your blood is drawn makes quite a difference in assessing the quantity of hormones circulating in your body. Hormonal levels fluctuate throughout the day in a rhythmic cycle called *diurnal variation*. Each woman will experience a different pattern of rising and falling. A single test of your hormones does not provide an accurate indication of what's really going on in your body. Your progesterone level may be high at noon, but it may drop sharply in the evening—precisely the time when you feel the most "draggy." Your testosterone levels may peak in the morning, and you find yourself reaching for your partner just as it's time to get up and go to work; but by evening, those levels might plummet, and you are mystified and disturbed to discover that you have lost interest in sex.

Most saliva tests are not one-shot deals but rather measure your hormonal fluctuations over a given period of time. This makes them far more accurate than blood tests. A salivary test can be conducted several times a day over the course of several days or weeks, depending on the particular lab you choose and the instructions of your physician. The results show the ebb and flow of your own unique hormonal patterns.

How Is the Saliva Test Performed?

At this time, the most comprehensive saliva tests are generally available through your health-care provider. Moreover, there is no single "saliva test." Different laboratories use different protocols.

- Some salivary tests involved taking a onetime sample by chewing gum or placing saliva in a test tube. They are less expensive than blood tests but otherwise are no different. They offer a one-shot-deal glimpse into your hormonal profile.
- More accurate salivary tests involve collecting samples over the course of time. This way you can see the ebb and flow of your hormones through the menstrual cycle. This is helpful even if you are postmenopausal, because your body still goes through cyclic phases and your hormones will not necessarily remain at the same levels all the time.

Both salivary tests are really very simple and can be carried out in the privacy of your home. Just chew the gum or spit into the test tube, seal the tube, and mail it to the lab. No fuss, no muss, no needles, no blood, no stress. Results are available to you and your doctor within a few days.

What Does the Saliva Test Show?

Saliva tests usually measure the five major sex steroid hormones—estrogen, progesterone, testosterone, cortisol, and DHEA. Generally speaking, most salivary tests will measure estradiol, while others may actually measure all three forms of estrogen (estriol, estrone, and estradiol). Each hormone is carefully charted so that you know its precise quantity at any given time of day over a sustained period of time. Your doctor will interpret the lab's report, analyzing the hormonal levels in your body to determine whether they are high or low, and when the fluctuations occur. Based on these findings, he or she will create a highly individualized hormone replacement program.

For example, let's say your estriol levels are low five days each month during the morning hours. You can receive a dosage of estradiol supplementation that precisely fills in what your body isn't producing on its own and precisely when your body isn't producing it. You are not being flooded with unnecessarily large quantities of estradiol that your body is unable to handle. You are receiving exactly what you need. And if you do need some estradiol, it can be administered in the exact quantity that you need, at the times of the month when you are deficient. This way your sensitive breast tissue is not flooded with unnecessary estradiol.

Your doctor may also repeat the test after a few months of treatment to assess whether the hormonal dose is correct and the imbalances have actually been rectified. Two women may have identical hormonal levels but may not respond in the same way to ostensibly identical treatment. Hormonal treatments should be adjusted, always in keeping with how *you* respond and with what is and is not called for in your body.

Creating a Safe HRT Program

Now that you and your doctor know exactly which hormonal levels are below the normal range in your body, you can begin a responsible HRT program.

My own bias would still be for you to take the information you have gleaned from the salivary test and begin by approaching your hormonal deficiencies using the herbs and supplements recommended in chapter 4. If you feel better using actual hormones, however, it is crucial that you and your physician use hormones that will help rather than injure your body. Here are some basic definitions and pointers.

What Are "Natural" Hormones?

Natural hormones are usually synthesized from soy or yam. They are superior to their less-than-natural counterparts because they are virtually identical to the hormones produced by your body. Natural estrogen, which is a derivative of soy, is more compatible with your hormone receptors than the horse-based product so often prescribed in conventional HRT. Natural progesterone, manufactured from wild yams or soy, is likewise a better match than synthetic progestin. Because these products are so similar to humanly produced hormones, they have fewer negative effects and are integrated by the body more smoothly.

Safe Estrogen Replacement

Safe estrogen replacement doesn't just concern the origin of the estrogen—horse based versus plant based. It also concerns the kind of estrogen being prescribed. Conventional estrogen replacement usually contains a large quantity of estradiol. Remember that this is the type of estrogen least desirable during and following menopause. Natural estrogen replacement, however, supplies estriol, which is the most desirable form of peri- and postmenopausal ERT. Tri-Est® is an example of an estrogen product that contains 80 percent estriol, 10 percent estrone, and only 10 percent estradiol. There are other similar products available. Clearly, these supply your body with the most useful and least destructive form of estrogen.

Progesterone Replacement

Natural progesterone is so similar to your body's own hormone that it's both effective and harmless to your body. If a salivary hormone test shows that you need progesterone replacement, my advice is that you use natural micronized progesterone. This product has been processed and refined into tiny crystals that are easily absorbed into your system.

Testosterone Replacement

An increasing number of physicians are becoming increasingly aware of the importance of testosterone replacement. Androgen therapy, as it is called, must be used cautiously because excessive quantities can lead to overgrowth of body hair and to other metabolic problems.

If a salivary hormone test shows low testosterone levels and the herbs and supplements recommended in chapter 4 haven't alleviated your symptoms, you can try testosterone replacement—with caution. "Natural" testosterone replacement is preferred and available by prescription only. Ask your physician to start you off on a very low dose, and see if it has an impact. Often a small quantity can make a big difference. I have found testosterone to be of greater benefit than either estrogen or progesterone in most cases.

Replacing What's Really Missing: Vera's Story

All too many physicians immediately assume that low estrogen levels cause a perimenopausal woman's complaints of hot flashes, fatigue, irritability, or diminished libido. They reflexively prescribe ERT without ascertaining whether low estrogen is actually the culprit in the woman's complaints. They fail to take into account the fact that estrogen is one of five sex steroid hormones, all of which go through significant fluctuations during the menopausal years.

Vera J, a fifty-two-year-old homemaker, sat shyly on my couch. "I'm uncomfortable about bringing this up," she began. "I started going through the 'change of life'—that's what my mother used to call it—a few years ago. I must have been about forty-eight or so. I've had my share of hot flashes and they've made me uncomfortable but I can live with them. My problem is—" She broke off and stared.

"Please go on," I encouraged her.

"My problem is that I don't enjoy sex anymore. It isn't only because of vaginal dryness. I just have no interest. My husband and I have always had a good marriage and a happy sex life together, but I haven't wanted to make love for three years. I go through the motions because I love him and I want him to be happy, but he can tell that my heart isn't in it."

"Have you talked to your doctor?" I wanted to know.

"My doctor put me on estrogen replacement three years ago when I first brought up this problem. But it hasn't helped."

I arranged for Vera to see a holistically oriented gynecologist who ordered a salivary hormone test. The test results showed that her estrogen levels were too high. Her testosterone levels, on the other hand, were abysmally low. The new gynecologist advised natural testosterone replacement therapy and within weeks, Vera and her husband were enjoying a passionate second honeymoon. She called me on her return, giggling like a schoolgirl. "I feel like a bride again," she confided. "I don't know how to thank you."

DHEA Replacement

DHEA is available in two over-the-counter forms at the health food store or compounded with other hormones by prescription only. Consult your health care provider regarding the form of DHEA most appropriate for your needs.

Available Forms of Natural HRT

Natural hormones are available in an array of different forms. These include oral capsules or tablets, cream, sublingual drops, lozenges, and even suppositories. Your physician may have a particular company with whom he or she regularly works. If not, you may need to go to a compounding pharmacy that will prepare a product tailor-made to your needs. You will find a list of pharmacies and guidelines in the Resources section of this book (page 195).

HRT Isn't a "One-Size-Fits-All"

As you can see, your hormones are as individual as you are. Just as there are no two people with identical fingerprints, so there are no two women who require the same hormonal regimen. Today's technology has made available to us a wide and wonderful range of choices that were unheard of in the generation of our mothers and grandmothers. Using these choices wisely will enable us to move toward and through menopause with health and energy. Precise and appropriate hormone replacement can turn menopause into the most productive and vigorous time you've ever enjoyed.

Finding a Physician Who Will Work with You

Since your first step in embarking upon an HRT program is finding a physician who can guide you through it, I'd like to offer a few words of advice on how to go about this. It may be more difficult than you think.

While saliva testing has been used in medical schools and research institutions for over three decades, it has only recently been introduced as a clinical test to be used by physicians in their day-to-day practice. Many doctors have not heard of it, and those who have might not be ready to incorporate it into their practice.

Begin with your own physician, if he or she is someone with whom you already have a rapport and whom you trust. I hope that this individual will be supportive and knowledgeable. If, however, you encounter resistance on your doctor's part, you will need to search for someone else. The Resources section (page 195) will help you to get started by supplying you with names of organizations that can refer you to physicians likely to be receptive to this approach.

You must be prepared to interview several doctors. Don't be surprised if you encounter some resistance from physicians who insist that this isn't "standard of care." It should be the standard of your care! In this day and age, there is no excuse for guesswork where hormones are concerned. Modern science has generated the technology to provide accurate and useful measures of hormonal levels, and it is your right as a patient to insist upon those measures before you put a single pill into your mouth!

If you find a doctor who is honest enough to admit that he or she is ignorant of salivary testing and open-minded enough to explore what it's all about and incorporate it into your treatment protocol, you can suggest some helpful books, journal articles, Web sites, and organizations. The Resources section at the end of this book (page 195) will provide you with further information. Make sure also that your physician is familiar with natural hormone replacement, because salivary hormone testing is just the beginning. Once you have determined which hormones should be augmented, your physician will need to guide you through the creation of your safe HRT program.

Eight

Putting It All Together

"How can I put this all together?" This is probably the question I hear most frequently from patients to whom I've outlined the total menopause program discussed in this book. These patients often react with dismay and even panic, afraid that they will be unable to put my recommendations into practice. Here's what I tell them: It may seem overwhelming, but it's not. You don't need to do a complete overhaul of your life. Just make the changes one step at a time.

This chapter is designed to help you break down the menopause program into manageable steps, based on your lifestyle, personal preferences, and medical profile. It will help you to set priorities and realistic goals so that you can really stick with the health-embracing changes you make. You will learn which questions to ask yourself and how answering these questions will assist you in creating a realistic, health-affirming program that really works for *you*.

Start Where You Are

Remember what I said in chapter 5 about setting up an exercise program? I told you that the first part of your body to exercise is your brain! That doesn't apply only to physical exercise but to all aspects of your menopausal program. The first and most important step toward health both during and after menopause will take place in your mind. You will need some quiet time, a pad, a pen—and all the brain power you can muster to engage in the careful and practical planning required.

Looking Ahead to Perimenopause

Some of you may not yet be going through perimenopause. Instead, you may be planning ahead. You would like to set the stage and prepare your body and your lifestyle for a change that still lies well in the future. Perhaps you are in your late thirties or early forties. Perhaps some of your friends are already beginning to experience symptoms that could be perimenopausal, or perhaps your mother or grandmother warned you that early menopause runs in the family, and you should be prepared.

If you're in this category—congratulations! You can get a head start on making lifestyle changes that will virtually guarantee you an easy passage through midlife. You can incorporate these important changes into your life in a gradual, leisurely way.

Since you don't know what perimenopausal discomforts—if any— you will experience, you should not begin a program of nutritional supplementation, beyond taking a multivitamin-multimineral supplement daily if you are not already doing so. I don't see much point in taking an herb like black cohosh, for example, preventively. There will be plenty of time to use this and other herbs if the symptoms present themselves.

What you *can* do now is change your dietary habits. Refer to chapter 3 (page 32) for a gradual, step-by-step program for modifying your diet and transforming it into a permanent, health-embracing lifestyle.

You can also begin to incorporate exercise into your weekly routine. Refer to chapter 5 (page 125) for a more complete discussion of how you can do this in a gradual and manageable fashion.

When you set up your exercise program, try to tailor it to your medical concerns and family history. If osteoporosis runs in your family, for example, you will want to start as early as possible on a weight-training program. If cardiovascular disease runs in your family, on the other hand, you will probably want to focus more of your attention on aerobic exercise. Of course, the final goal is to engage in both forms of exercise on a regular and sustained basis.

It won't hurt you to supplement with herbs if you're concerned about such issues as osteoporosis or cardiovascular disease. Supplements such as ipriflavone, for example, won't hurt you to use preventively. The same is true for vitamin E and CoQ_{10}. In fact, I'd advise you to get a jump start on supplementation if these problems run in your family—unless you are blessed with designer genes that protect you against conditions that have affected your other family members. Consult chapter 4 for a more thorough discussion of supplements that prevent these illnesses.

Once you have reached perimenopause, I hope that you will be in very good physical and emotional shape. You will have set the stage for the easiest and smoothest possible menopausal transition. Discomforts may, however, arise. The next section will teach you how to approach them.

So You're Perimenopausal

Many of you are reading this book because you have already started perimenopause and are experiencing discomforts. Perhaps these discomforts are disrupting your life to the extent that it seems doubly overwhelming to plan out long-term lifestyle changes. What you're looking for is relief—and the sooner the better!

Start by making a list of your concerns. Are you experiencing perimenopausal symptoms now? If so, which ones? Of the most common complaints—hot flashes, fatigue, irritability, forgetfulness, vaginal dryness, and insomnia—which is/are the most troublesome to you?

Let's say you are experiencing hot flashes. They're driving you crazy. You're also tired and lose concentration easily. Begin with nutritional supplementation—specifically, black cohosh. It should provide you with rapid relief. If black cohosh isn't sufficient to alleviate your discomforts, then follow the herbal regimen outlined in chapter 4, experimenting until you have found a formula that gives you some respite.

Use your newfound mental clarity and physical energy to create a realistic plan to modify your diet and incorporate some exercise into your lifestyle. The suggestions in chapters 3 and 5 will help you to do this.

If you remain symptomatic even after trying herbal remedies, dietary modifications, and a regular exercise regimen, you may wish to consult a physician. He or she can help you to assess whether your hormones are at normal levels and, if not, which particular hormones require replacement. A physician will also help you rule out other disorders—such as thyroid problems—that often masquerade as perimenopausal complaints.

If you require hormone replacement, use the suggestions in chapter 7 to guide you through a safe hormonal therapy program.

At every stage of the process, your attitude will make a crucial difference in your ability to move from discomfort to physical health and vitality. Persistent physical symptoms can often be the sign of unresolved emotional issues or simply of an excessively stressful lifestyle. The most nutritious diet, rigorous exercise program, and carefully constructed herbal regimen will not be optimally successful if you are not getting enough rest, lead a hurried and high-pressure life, or are burdened by worries and fears.

So take a little time to take stock of your life. Are you getting enough sleep? Do you give yourself time for recreation? Are you nurturing yourself and your important relationships? Can you make any changes in schedule, employment, or some other area of your life that will reduce the stress you may be currently experiencing?

Is anything worrying you? Use chapter 6 to assist you in understanding some of the issues that most commonly concern perimenopausal women. Chapter 6 will also help you to figure out whether you need professional help in dealing with your distress—and, if so, what kind of help and how to locate it.

Of course, you should adapt all these steps, whether practical or emotional, to your own particular needs and preferences. Let's say you love to cook and your life revolves around the stove and the dinner table. You may find dietary modifications both challenging and fun, and they may be the first component of your menopausal program that you decide to implement. Later, once you have incorporated dietary changes into your life, you can begin to look at increasing the amount of exercise you get or at obtaining some herbs from the health food store.

On the other hand, if you are experiencing marital problems, you may want to begin with some first aid for your marriage. Perhaps all you need is a recharge, and a long romantic weekend is in order. Perhaps you need to assess your lifestyle together and restructure your time so that you can focus additional attention on each other. If your problems are more deep-seated, you may require some individual or joint counseling. Once you feel a little less overwhelmed by an emotionally draining situation, you can attend to your physical health.

Of course, it's best to approach any problem multi-modally—in other words, using many different types of therapeutic modalities at the same time. It stands to reason that the more healthful changes you can make, the more your health will improve. But it's not absolutely essential for you to approach your menopausal multi-modally. It would be better for you to take your changes slowly, step by step, so that you feel in control of the process, and so that the changes you make are permanent.

If You Are Postmenopausal

If you have already gone through the menopausal transition, your concerns are likely to be different from those of a woman going through perimenopause. You are probably past the stage of hot flashes and night sweats. You are probably focusing on more general issues of aging—particularly osteoporosis and cardiovascular disease.

Again, my advice is to begin where you are. Start by looking at your personal and family history. If osteoporosis runs in your family, for example, you will want to begin by emphasizing the components of the menopausal program that address osteoporosis. Start with nutritional supplementation and weight-training exercises. As you look toward modifying your diet, concentrate on adding the bone-building foods listed in chapter 3. All the other dietary recommendations—foods to eat and foods to avoid—can be implemented later.

If cardiovascular disease runs in your family, on the other hand, you should immediately begin creating a sensible and realistic aerobic exercise program, using the suggestions in chapter 5. Dietary changes will be critical to good health, so your next step should be a careful assessment of your diet with an eye to eliminating the "unhealthy" fats and substituting the "healthy" ones. The other dietary changes will follow afterward. Finally, you should start using herbs—such as garlic—that are known to reduce cholesterol levels and preserve cardiovascular health.

Reducing the Risk of Cancer

Because cancer strikes individuals of all ages, I have not listed it as either a perimenopausal or a postmenopausal concern. It would be remiss of me, however, if I didn't devote some attention to this alarming illness. Incidence of cancer is very much on the rise in this country, with the most recent statistics estimating that a third of the American population will suffer from cancer at some point in their lives.

Postmenopausal women are particularly vulnerable to certain cancers, such as those that affect the breasts and ovaries. If breast cancer runs in your family, you should aggressively implement the dietary modifications outlined in chapter 3. Since numerous studies have connected a low-fat, high-vegetable diet with cancer reduction, creating a diet that meets those criteria should be the first order of the day. Additionally, you should take herbs and nutritional supplements that are known to reduce the risk of cancer. These are listed in chapter 4 (page 64).

Although these healthful measures don't constitute a *guarantee* that you won't get cancer—cancer can strike people regardless of age, lifestyle, or other circumstances—you can certainly reduce your risk significantly. The better your overall health, the stronger your body and your immune system will be. Strength in these areas will enable you to combat cancer, as well as other diseases. Basic steps include quitting smoking if you are a smoker, getting enough exercise and rest, following a healthy diet, and limiting exposure to chemicals and toxins in the environment and in food. Since some studies have linked cancer with emotional stress and repressed negative feelings, the more you can learn to relax, the more you give yourself the extra edge against this disease.

The Best Is Yet to Come

We all march to the beat of our own drummers, as Henry David Thoreau once put it. We are highly individual in our needs, wants, and lifestyles. Our menopause programs, then, are going to be equally unique and individualized. This book has been designed to give you the building blocks of good menopausal health. How you implement these changes and tailor them to your unique needs will be up to you.

Remember that time is on your side. Menopause does not happen suddenly. Rather, it is a transition that takes place over many years. You have time in which to move gently toward a lifestyle that embraces good menopausal health. Use that time well. Don't make dramatic resolutions or drastic changes. It is better to take it slow and make fewer changes that will last than to rush into a whirlwind of activity that you are unable to sustain. The most perfect, health-centered lifestyle won't help you at all if you give it up. But a single change—let's say, incorporating exercise into your daily or weekly routine—can make a substantial difference to your health if you continue this practice for a lifetime.

This program is eminently workable. If you follow its guidelines, you will move through and beyond menopause feeling vigorous and healthy. In fact, I'll bet that you will actually be healthier than you were before you started out! You can enjoy more vitality and joie de vivre than you've ever known. You will have all the benefits of a senior—extra freedom, extra time, and a storehouse of accumulated life wisdom—without the dreaded age-related physical drawbacks so many people believe are inevitable. You can be more vigorous and energetic than you were when you were thirty.

It is my conviction that some of the youth worship that abounds in our society will begin to abate and change in the coming decades. According to conservative government figures from 1996, the number of Americans over age sixty-five will more than double between the years 2000 and 2050, reaching an unprecedented 80 million. We are poised on the cusp of a new era in which all of American society will forced to examine its beliefs about aging. This is the perfect time for you to reassess your own attitudes toward menopause and aging, and to learn how to regard the changes in your body in a positive light.

The best years of your life are just beginning.

Selected References

There is a vast number of scientific studies, articles, and books devoted to each of the subjects covered in *How to Stop the Menopausal Roller Coaster.* Obviously, an exhaustive compendium lies beyond the purview of this book. It is my hope that the Selected References below will give you an idea of the formidable amount of evidence supporting the approaches I've recommended. If you want additional information about any of these topics, you can continue your own investigation using some of the Suggestions for Further Reading.

Chapter 1: Understanding Menopause: Is Menopause a Disease?

Liebert, M.A. Natural intervention for menopause. *Women's Health Alternative Medicine Report* 1, no. 1 (1999):1–4.

Mayo, J.L. A natural approach to menopause. *Clinical Nutrition Insights* 5, no. 7 (July 1997):1–8.

Rutlege, J.C., Hyson, D.A., Garduno D., et al. Lifestyle modification program in management of patients with coronary artery disease. *J Cardiopulm Rehab* 19, no. 4 (1999):226–34.

Taffe, A.M, and Cuffield, J. "Natural" hormone replacement therapy and dietary supplements used in the treatment of menopausal symptoms. *Lippincott's Primary Care Physician* 2, no. 3 (1998):292–302.

Chapter 2: Hormone Replacement Therapy: Pros and Cons

General Discussion of Hormone Replacement Therapy

Kessel, B. Alternatives to estrogen for menopausal women. *Proceedings of the Society of Experimental Biological Medicine* 217, no. 1 (1998):38–44.

Soffia, V.M., Alternatives to hormone replacement for menopause. *Alternative Therapies* 2, no. 2 (1996):34–39.

Taylor, M. Alternatives to conventional hormone replacement therapy. *Complementary Therapies* 23, no. 8 (1997):514–32.

General Discussion of HRT

Girdler, S.S., O'Briant, C., and Steege, J. A comparison of the effect of estrogen with or without progesterone on mood and physical symptoms in postmenopausal women. *Journal of Women's Health and Gender-Based Medicine* 8, no. 5 (1999):637ff.

Greendale, G.A., Reboussin, B.A., Hogan, P., et al. Symptom relief and side effects of postmenopausal hormones: results from the postmenopausal estrogen/progestin interventions trial. *Obstet Gynecol* 98 (1998):982–88.

Hogervorst, E., Boshusen, M., and Riedel, W. 1998 Curt P. Richter Award: The effect of hormone replacement therapy on cognitive function in elderly women. *Psychoneuroendocrin* 21, no. 1 (1999):43–68.

Pearce, M.J., and Hauton, K. Psychological and sexual aspects of menopause and hormone replacement therapy. *Bailliere Clinic Obstets and Gynecol* 10, no. 3 (1996):385–99.

Shaywitz, S.E., Shaywitz, A.B., Pugh, K.R., et al. Effect of estrogen on brain activation patterns in postmenopausal women during working memory tasks. *JAMA* 281, no. 13 (1999):1197–1202.

HRT and Osteoporosis

Eiken, P., Kolthoff, N., and Sielsen, S.P. Effect of 10 years' HRT on bone mineral content in postmenopausal women. *Bone* Suppl. 5 (1996): 191S–93S.

Hailey, D., Sampietro-Colom, L., Marshall, D., et al. The effectiveness of bone density measurement and associated treatments for the prevention of fractures. *International Journal of Technological Assessment of Healthcare* 14, no. 2 (1998):237–54.

Hart, D.M., Farish, E., Fletcher, C.D., et al. Long-term effects of continuous hormone replacement therapy on bone turnover and lipid metabolism in postmenopausal women. *Osteoporosis Intl* 4, no. 4 (1998):326–32.

Kanis, J.A. Estrogens, the menopause, and osteoporosis. *Bone* Suppl. 5 (1996): 185S–90S.

Rosenberg, S., Gevers, R., Peretz, A., et al. Decrease of bone mineral density during estrogen substitution therapy. *Maturitas* 17, no. 3 (1993):205–10.

Samsiol, G. Osteoporosis—an update. *Acta Obstet Gynecol Scandinavia* 76, no. 3 (1997):189–99.

Sener, A.B., Seckin, N.C., Ozaren, S., et al. The effects of HRT on uterine fibroids in postmenopausal women. *Fertil Steril* 65, no. 2 (1996):354–57.

HRT and Cardiovascular Disease

Hulley, S., Grady, D., Buah, T., et al. Randomized trial of estrogen plus progestin for secondary prevention of coronary heart disease in postmenopausal women. *JAMA* 280, no. 7 (1998):605–13.

Miller, V.T., Barnabei, V., Kessler, C., et al. Effects of estrogen or estrogen/progestin regimens on heart disease risk factors in postmenopausal women. *JAMA* 273, no. 3 (1995):199–208.

Perez, G.S., Rodriguez, L.A., Castellsague, J., et al. Hormone replacement therapy and risk of venous thromboembolism: population based case-control study. *BMJ* 314 (1997):796–800.

Rodstrom, K., Bengtsoon, C., Lissner, L., et al. Pre-existing risk factor profiles in users and non-users of hormone replacement therapy. *BMJ* 318 (1999): 890–93.

HRT and Cancer

Colditz, G.A. Relationship between estrogen levels, use of hormone replacement therapy, and breast cancer. *J Nat Can Inst* 90, no. 11 (1998):34–43.

Collaborative Group on Hormonal Factors in Breast Cancer. Breast cancer and hormone replacement therapy: collaborative reanalysis of date from 51 epidemiological studies of 52,705 women with breast cancer and 108,705 women without breast cancer. *Lancet* 350, no. 9084 (1997):1047–59.

Gapstur, S.M., Morrow, M., and Sellers, T.A. Hormone replacement therapy and risk of breast cancer with a favorable histology. *JAMA* 281 (1999):2091–97.

Pritchard, K.I. Estrogen/hormone replacement therapy and the etiology of breast cancer. *Rec Res Canc Res* 152 (1998):22–31.

Rodrigues, C., Calle, E.E., Coates, R.J., et al. Estrogen replacement therapy and fatal ovarian cancer. *Am Jour of Epidemiol* 141, no. 9 (1995):828–35.

Schairer, C., Lubin, J., Troisi, R., et al. Menopausal estrogen and estrogen-progestin replacement therapy and breast cancer risk. *JAMA* 283, no. 4 (2000):485–91.

Tavani, A., and LaVecchia, C. The adverse effects of hormone replacement therapy. *Drugs Aging* 14, no. 5 (1999):347–57.

Noncompliance with HRT Regimens

Doren, M., and Schneider, H.P. Long-term compliance of continuous combination estrogen and progestogen in postmenopausal women. *Maturitas* 25, no. 2 (1996):99–105.

Faulkner, D.C., Young, C., Hutchins, D., et al. Patient noncompliance with HRT: a nationwide estimate using a large prescription database. *Menopause* 5, no. 4 (1998):226–29.

Chapter 3: Diet:
Your Best Hormone Replacement Therapy

Soybeans, Phytoestrogens, and Menopause

Albertazzi, P., Pansini, F., Bottazzi, G., et al. Dietary soy supplementation and phytoestrogen levels. *Obstet Gynecol* 92, no. 2 (August 1999):229–31.

Clarkson, T.B., Anthony, M.S., Williams, J.K., et al. The potential of soybean phytoestrogens for postmenopausal hormone replacement therapy. *Proc Soc Exp Biol Med* 271, no. 3 (1998):365–68.

Goodman, M.T., Wilkens, L.R., Hankin, J.H., et al. Association of soy and fiber consumption with the risk of endometrial cancer. *Am J Epidemiol* 146, no. 4 (1997):294–306.

Humfrey, C.D. Phytoestrogens and human health effects: weighing up the current evidence. *Nat Tox* 6, no. 2 (1998):51–59.

Ingram, D., Sanders, K., Kolybaba, M., et al. Case-control study of phyto-estrogens and breast cancer. *Lancet* 350 (1997):990–94.

Lock, M. Contested meanings of menopause. *Lancet* 337 (1991): 1270–72.

Reichert, R.G. Phyto-estrogens. *Quarterly Review of Natural Medicine* (spring 1994):27–33.

Washburn, S., Burke, G.L., Morgan, T., et al. Effect of soy protein supplementation on serum lipoproteins, blood pressure, and menopausal symptoms in perimenopausal women. *Menopause* 6, no. 1 (1999):7–13.

The Impact of Diet on Good Health

Baghurst, P.A., and Rohan, T.E. High-fiber diets and reduced risk of breast cancer. *Int J Cancer* 56, no. 2 (1994): 173–76.

Bradlow, H.L., Michnovicz, J.J., Halper, M., et al. Long-term responses of women to indole-3-carbinol or a high fiber diet. *Cancer Epidemiol Markers* 3, no. 7 (1994):591–95.

Dorgan, J.F., Reichman, M.E., Judd, J.T., et al. Relation of energy, fat, and fiber intakes to plasma concentrations of estrogens and androgens in premenopausal women. *Am J Clin Nutrition* 64 (1996):25–31.

Fernandez, E., Chatenoud, L., LaVecchia, C., et al. Fish consumption and cancer risk. *Am J Clin Nutrition* 79 (1999):85–90.

Food, Nutrition and Prevention of Cancer: A Global Perspective. Washington, D.C.: American Institute for Cancer Research, 1997.

Holmes, M.D., Hunter, D.J., Colditz, G.A., et al. Association of dietary intake of fat and fatty acids with risk of breast cancer. *JAMA* 281, no. 10 (1999):914–20.

Hoyer, A.P., et al. Pesticides and breast cancer. *Lancet* 351 (1998): 1816–20.

Muhlbauer, R.C., and Li, F. Effects of vegetables on bone metabolism. *Nature* (1999):343–44.

Stoll, B.A. Breast cancer and the western diet: the role of fatty acids and antioxidant vitamins. *Eur J Cancer* 34, no. 12 (1998):1852–56.

Tognoni, G. Fish oil supplements and cardiac disease. Address presented to the American College of Cardiology, March 11, 1999.

Wu, A.H., Pike, M.C., and Stram, D.O. Meta-analysis: dietary fat intake, serum estrogen levels, and the risk of breast cancer. *J Nat Cancer Inst* 91, no. 6 (1999):529–34.

Chapter 4: Nutritional Supplements to Help You Avoid the Roller Coaster

Vitamins and Minerals

Adams, A.K., Wermuth, E.O., McBride, P.E. Antioxidant vitamins and the prevention of coronary heart disease. *Am Fam Phys* 60, no. 3 (1999):895–904.

Benefits of Nutritional Supplements. Washington, D.C.: Council for Responsible Nutrition, 1993.

Benner, S.E., et al. Clinical chemoprevention: developing a cancer prevention strategy. *J Natl Cancer Inst* 85, no. 18 (1993):1446–47.

Chait, A., Malinow, M.R., Nevin, D.N., et al. Increased dietary micronutrients decrease serum homocysteins concentration in patients at high risk of cardiovascular disease. *Am J Clin Nutr* 70, no. 5 (1999):881–87.

Fugh-Berman, A., Cott, J.M. Dietary supplements and natural products as psychotherapeutic agents. *Psychosom Med* 61, no. 5 (1999):712–28.

Keller, C., Fullerton, J., and Mobley, C. Supplements and complementary alternatives to HRT. *J Am Acad Nurse Pract* 11, no. 5 (1999):187–98.

Lechance, Pa. To supplement or not to supplement: is it a question? *Am J Coll Nutr* 13, no. 2 (1994):113–15.

Mayne, S.T., et al. Dietery beta carotene and lung cancer risk in U.S. nonsmokers. *J Natl Canc Inst* 86, no. 1 (1994):33–38.

Safety of Vitamins and Minerals: A Summary of the Findings of Key Nutrients. Washington, D.C.: Council for Responsible Nutrition, 1991.

Seibel, M.M. The role of nutrition and nutritional supplements in women's health. *Fertil Steril* 72, no. 4 (1999):579–91.

Verlangiere, A.J., Bush, M.J. Effects of d-alpha-tocopherol supplementation on experimentally induced primate atherosclerosis. *J Am Coll Nutr* 11, no. 2 (1992):131–38.

Nutritional Supplements

Head, K.A. Ipriflavone: an important bone-building isoflavone. *Altern Med Rev* 4, no. 1 (1999):10–22.

Hoppe, U., Bugemann, J., Diembeck, W., et al. Coenzyme Q_{10}, a cutaneous antioxidant and energizer. *Biofactors* 9, nos. 2–4 (1999):371–78.

Isihara, M. Effect of gamma oryzanol on serum lipid peroxide level and climacteric disturbances. *Asia-Oceania J Obstet Gynaecol* 10, no. 3 (1984):317.

Lieberman, S. Ipriflavone: A natural alternative for the treatment of osteoporosis. *Women's Health Alternative Medicine Report* 1, no. 6 (1999):1–3.

Schreiber, M.D., and Rebar, R.W. Ipriflavones and postmenopausal bone health—a viable alternative to estrogen therapy? *Menopause* 6, no. 3 (1999):233–41.

Herbal Supplements

Barrett, B., Kofer, D., and Rubapo, D. Assessing the risks and benefits of herbal medicines: an overview of scientific evidence. *Altern Ther Health Med* 5, no. 4 (1999):40–49.

Kidd, P.M. A review of nutrients and botanicals in the integrative management of cognitive dysfunction. *Altern Med Rev* 4, no. 3 (1999):144–61.

Lieberman, S. Nutraceutical review of St. John's Wort (*Hypericum perforatum*) for the treatment of depression. *Journal of Women's Health* 7, no. 7 (1998):177–82.

———. A review of the effectiveness of *Cimifuga racemosa* (black cohosh) for the symptoms of menopause. *Journal of Women's Health* 7, no. 5 (1998):525–29.

Punnonen, R., and Lukola, A. Oestrogenlike effects of ginseng. *Br Med Jour* 281 (1980):1110.

Warshafsky, S., Kamer, R.S., and Sivak, S.L. The effect of garlic on total serum cholesterol: a meta-analysis. *Annals Int Med* 119 (1993):599–605.

Weed, S.S. Menopause and beyond: the wise woman way. *J Nurse Midwifery* 44, no. 3 (1999):267–79.

Chapter 5: Incorporating Exercise into Your Menopausal Program

General Benefits of Exercise

Burghardt, M. Exercise at menopause: A critical difference. *Medscape Women's Health* 4, no. 1 (1999):1.

Rockhill, B., Willett, W.C., and Hunter, D.J., et al. A prospective study of recreational physical activity and breast cancer risk. *Arch Intern Med* 159 (1999):2290–96.

Exercise and Cardiovascular Disease

Belardinelli, R., Geogiou, D., Cianci, C., et al. Randomized controlled trial of long-term moderate exercise training in chronic heart failure. *Circulation* 99, no. 9 (1999):1773–82.

Mensink, G., Ziese, T., and Kok, F.J. Benefits of leisure-time physical activity on the cardiovascular risk profile at older age. *Int Jour Epidemiol* 28 (1999):659–66.

Exercise and Mental Health

Blumenthal, J.A., Babyak, M.A., and Moore, K.A. Effects of exercise training on older patients with major depression. *Arch Intern Med* 159 (1999):2349–56.

DiLorenzo, T.M., Bargman, E.P., Stucky-Ropp, R., et al. Long-term effects of aerobic exercise on psychological outcomes. *Prev Med* 28, no. 1 (1999):75–85.

Exercise and Osteoporosis

Bemden, D.A. Exercise interventions for osteoporosis prevention in post-menopausal women. *J Okla State Med Assoc* 92, no. 2 (1999):66–70.

Berard, A., Bravo, G., and Gauthies, P. Meta-analysis of the effectiveness of physical exercise for prevention of bone loss in postmenopausal women. *Osteop Int* 7, no. 4 (1997):331–37.

Layne, J.E., and Nelson, M.E. The effects of progressive resistance training on bone density: a review. *Med Sci Sports Exerc* 3 (1999):25–30.

Sheth, O. Osteoporosis and exercise: A review. *Mt Sinai J Med* 66, no. 3 (1999):197–200.

Chapter 6: Attitude and Emotions During Menopause

Byles, J. A positive view of older women. *Aust N Z J Public Health* 22, no. 7 (1998):743–45.

Gannon, L., and Stevens, J. Portraits of menopause in the mass media. *Women's Health* 27, no. 3 (1998):1–15.

Gimbel, M.A. Yoga, meditation and imagery—clinical applications. *Nurse Pract Forum* 9, no. 4 (1998):243–55.

Harmon, R.L., and Myers, M.A. Prayer and meditation as medical therapies. *Phys Med Rehab Clin N Am* 10, no. 3 (1999):651–62.

Hausdorff, J.M., Levy, B.R., and Wei, J.Y. The power of ageism on physical function in older persons. *J Am Geriatr Soc* 47 (1999):1–4.

Kennedy, M. Growing old doesn't mean growing ill. *WMJ* 97, no. 11 (1998):28–29.

Linney, B.J. How to be viewed as a sage in your elder years. *Physician Exec* 25, no. 2 (1999):68–79.

Loehr, J., Verma, S., and Seguin, R. Issues of sexuality in older women. *Journal of Women's Health* 6, no. 4 (1997):451–57.

Marsiglio, W., and Donnelly, D. Sexual relations in later life: a national study of married persons. *J Gerontol* 46, no. 6 (1991):S339–44.

Meddin, J.R. Dimensions of spiritual meaning and well-being in the lives of ten older Australians. *Int J Aging Hum Dev* 47, no. 3 (1998):163–75.

Schotanus, W.M. Healthy aging: the body/mind/spirit connection. *J Med Assoc Ga* 86, no. 2 (1997):127–28.

Travis, F., and Wallace, R.K. Autonomic and EEG practices during eyes-closed rest and Transcendental Meditation practice. *Conscious Cogn* 8, no. 3 (1999):302–18.

Webb, L., Delaney, J.J., and Young, L.R. Age, interpersonal attraction, and social interaction. *Res Aging* 11, no. 1 (1989):107–23.

Yasgur, B.S. Menopausal women: older, wiser and happier too. *OBG Management* 21 (November 1999):21.

Chapter 7: HRT Revisited—Safely

Arit, W. DHEA. *N Engl J Med* 341 (1999):1013–20.

Boschert, S. Progesterone cream soothes vasomotor ills. *Ob Gyn News*, January 1, 1999:11.

Ellison, P. Measurement of salivary progesterone. *Annals of the New York Academy of Sciences* (1992):161–76.

Hargrove, J.T., and Oseen, K.G. An alternative method of hormone replacement therapy using the natural sex steroid hormones. *Menopause* 6 (1995):653–74.

Lipson, S., and Ellison, P. Development of protocols for the application of salivary steroid analysis to field conditions. *Am J Hum Biol* 1 (1989):249–55.

Sarrel, P. Androgens and sexual function. *J Reprod Med* 43, no. 10 (1998):847–56.

Yasgur, B.S. Thyroid: the missing T in HRT. *OBG Management* (March 1999):87.

Yen, S., Morales, A.J., and Khorram, O. Replacement of DHEA in aging men and women: potential remedial effects. *Annals of the New York Academy of Sciences* 774 (1995):128–42.

Suggestions for Further Reading

Ahlgrimm, Marla, and John M. Kells. *The HRT Solution: Optimizing Your Hormone Potential*. Garden City Park, N.Y.: Avery Publishing Group, 1999.

Appleton, N. *Healthy Bones: What You Should Know About Osteoporosis*. Garden City Park, N.Y.: Avery Publishing Group, 1991: 84–88.

Balch, James F., and Phyllis A. Balch. *Prescription for Nutritional Healing*. Garden City Park, N.Y.: Avery Publishing Group, 1990.

Benson, Herbert. *The Relaxation Response*. New York: Morrow/Avon Books, 2000.

Borysenko, Joan. *Minding the Body, Mending the Mind*. Reading, Mass.: Addison-Wesley, 1987.

Brown, Donald. *Herbal Prescriptions for Better Health*. Rocklin, Calif.: Prima Publishing, 1996.

Colbin, Annemarie. *Food and Healing*. New York: Ballantine, 1996.

———. *Food and Our Bones*. New York: Plume, 1998.

DeMarco, Carolyn. *Take Charge of Your Body*. Portland, Or.: Powells Books, 1995.

Germains, Carl. *The Osteoporosis Solution*. New York: Kensington Books, 1999.

Goldberg, Burton. *Alternative Medicine Guide to Women's Health*. Puyallup, Wash.: Future Medicine Publishing, 1998.

Greenberg, Patricia, et al. *175 Delicious, Nutritious, Easy-to-Prepare Recipes Featuring Tofu, Tempeh, and Various Forms of Nature's Healthiest Bean*. New York: Random House, 1998.

Hooton, Claire. *Tai Chi for Beginners: Ten Minutes of Health and Fitness*. New York: Berkley, 1996.

Hudson, Tori. *Women's Encyclopedia of Natural Medicine*. Los Angeles: Keats Publishing, 1999.

Ikenze, Ifeoma. *Menopause and Homeopathy: A Guide for Women in Midlife*. Berkeley: North Atlantic Books, 1999.

Kaptchuk, Ted. *The Web That Has No Weaver: Understanding Chinese Medicine*. Lincolnwood, Ill.: NTC/Contemporary Publishing, 2000.

LeShan, Lawrence. *How to Meditate*. New York: Bantam, 1984.

Lieberman, Shari. *The Real Vitamin and Mineral Book*. Garden City Park, N.Y.: Avery Publishing Group, 1997.

Liu, Hong. *The Healing Art of Qi Gong*. New York: Warner, 1999.

Lonsdorf, Nancy, et al. *A Woman's Best Medicine: Health, Happiness and Long Life Through Maharishi Ayur-veda*. New York: Jeremy P. Tarcher, 1995.

Northrup, Christiane. *Women's Bodies, Women's Wisdom*. New York: Bantam, 1994.

Ojeda, Linda. *Menopause Without Medicine*. Alameda, Calif.: Hunter House, 1995.

Ransohoff, Rita M. *Venus After Forty: Sexual Myths, Men's Fantasies, and Truths About Middle-Aged Women*. Far Hills, N.J.: New Horizons Press, 1987.

Sass, Lorna J. *The New Soy Cookbook: Tempting Recipes for Soybeans, Soy Milk, Tofu, Tempeh, Miso, and Soy Sauce*. San Fransisco: Chronicle Books, 1998.

Schiffman, Erich. *Yoga—The Spirit and Practice of Moving Into Stillness*. New York: Simon and Schuster, 1996.

Scialli, Anthony (ed.). *The National Women's Health Resource Center Book of Women's Health*. New York: Morrow, 1999.

Stones, Lee, and Michael Stones. *Sex May Be Wasted on the Young*. North York, Ontario: Captus Press, 1996.

Weed, Susun S. *Menopausal Years*. Woodstock, N.Y.: Ash Tree Publishing, 1992.

Woodruff, Sandra. *Secrets of Cooking for Long Life*. Garden City Park, N.Y.: Avery Publishing Group, 1999.

Wright, Jonathan, and John Morgenthaler. *Natural Hormone Replacement: For Women over 45*. Petaluma, Calif.: Smart Publications, 1997.

Resources

The purpose of this section is to give you some leads as to how you can obtain the types of products or services mentioned in this book. Please understand that I'm not trying to provide you with an exhaustive list of the item in question. I'm merely trying to get you started. And please remember that no two people will respond to a given approach or remedy the same way. You will have to experiment for yourself.

Organizations

Note: Please be aware that addresses and telephone numbers may be subject to change.

Aging, Menopause, and General Women's Health

A Friend Indeed
Box 1710
Champlain, NY 11219-1710
(514) 843-5730
Fax (514) 843-5681

Alliance for Aging Research
2021 K Street NW, Suite 305
Washington, DC 20006
(202) 293-2856

A Woman's Time
Dr. Tori Hudson
2067 NW Lovejoy
Portland, OR 97209
(503) 222-2322

National Council on the Aging, Inc.
409 Third Street SW
Washington, DC 20024
(202) 479-1200
TID (202) 479-6674

National Institute on Aging
31 Center Drive, MSC 2292
Bethesda, MD 20892
(301) 496-1752

National Organization for Women
733 Fifteenth Street NW
Washington, DC 20005
(202) 628-8669

National Women's Health Network
1325 G Street NW
Washington, DC 20005
(202) 347-1140

National Women's Health Resource Center
2440 M Street NW, Suite 201
Washington, DC 20037
(202) 293-6045

North American Menopause Society
University Hospitals/Department of Obstetrics and Gynecology
2074 Abington Road
Cleveland, OH 44106
Fax (216) 844-3348
Written requests only.

Older Women's League (OWL)
333 Eleventh Street NW, Suite 700
Washington, DC 20001
(202) 783-6686

Cancer

Cancer Control Society (Alternative Cancer Treatment Resources)
2043 North Berendo
Los Angeles, CA 90027
(323) 663-7801

CanHelp (Alternative Cancer Resources)
3111 Paradise Bay Road
Port Ludlow, WA 98365-9771
(360) 437-2291

Exceptional Cancer Patients, Inc. (ECaP)
300 Plaza Middlesex
Middletown, CT 06456
(860) 343-5950

National Alliance of Breast Cancer Organizations
9 East 37th Street
New York, NY 10016
(212) 889-0606

National Cancer Institute
Cancer Information Service
9000 Rockville Pike
Bethesda, MD 20892
(800) 4-CANCER
(800) 422-6237

Y-ME
National Institute for Breast Cancer Information and Support
18220 Harwood Avenue
Homewood, IL 60430
(708) 799-8338

Cardiovascular Disease

American Heart Association
7320 Greenville Avenue
Dallas, TX 75321
(214) 373-6300

National Heart, Lung, and Blood Institute
9000 Rockville Pike
Bethesda, MD 20892
(301) 496-4236

Osteoporosis

National Osteoporosis Foundation
2100 M Street NW, Suite 602
Washington, DC 20037
(202) 223-2237

Nutrition and Food Safety

Center for Science in the Public Interest (Food Safety)
1875 Connecticut Avenue NW, Suite 300
Washington, DC 20009-5728
(202) 332-9110

Certification Board for Nutrition Specialists (Nutrition)
301 East 17th Street
New York, NY 10003
(212) 777-1037

Herbs

American Botanical Council
POB 12006
Austin, TX 78711
(512) 331-8868

American Herb Association
POB 1673
Nevada City, CA 95959

American Herbalists Guild
POB 746555
Arvada, CO 80006
(303) 423-8800

Herb Research Foundation
1007 Pearl Street
Boulder, CO 80302
(303) 449-2265

Referrals to Mental Health Professionals

American Psychological Association (APA)
750 First Street NE
Washington, DC 20002
(202) 336-5500

National Association of Social Workers (NASW)
750 First Street NE
Washington, DC 20002
(202) 408-8600

Personal Growth Programs and Support Groups

Al-Anon Family Services Group
1600 Corporate Landing Parkway
Virginia Beach, VA 23454

Alcoholics Anonymous (AA) Worldwide Services
Box 459
Grand Central Station, NY 10163
(212) 870-3400

The Omega Institute
150 Lake Drive
Rhinebeck, NY 12572
(914) 266-4444

The Option Institute and Fellowship
2080 South Undermountain Road
Sheffield, MA 01257
(413) 229-2100

The Option Method Network
Gary Skow
17681 Bruce Avenue
Monte Sereno, CA 95030
(408) 395-3286

Silva Method
1407 Calle Del Norte
P.O. Box 2249
Laredo, TX 78044-2249
(800) 545-6436

Zen Center
POB 91
Mountain View, CA 94042
(415) 966-1057

Compounding Pharmacies

Apothecure
1370 Midway Road
Dallas, TX 75244
(800) 969-6601

Bajamar Women's Health Care
9609 Dielman Rock Island
St. Louis, MO 63132
(800) 255-8025

Belmar Pharmacy
8015 West Alamed Avenue
Lakewood, CO 80226
(800) 525-9473

International Academy of Compounding Pharmacists
POB 1365
Sugarland, TX 77487
(713) 933-8400
(900) 927-4227

Lloyd Center Pharmacy
1302 Lloyd Center
Portland, OR 97232
(800) 358-8974

Women's International Pharmacy
5708 Monono Drive
Madison, WI 53716
(800) 279-5708

Nutritional, Herbal, and Homeopathic Companies

Avena Botanicals
219 Mill Street
Rockland, ME 04856
(207) 594-0694

Eclectic Institute
14385 SE Lusted Road
Sandy, OR 97055
(800) 332-4372

Enzymatic Therapies
825 Challenger Drive
Green Bay, WI 54311
(800) 783-2286

For Women Only
Dr. Shari Lieberman
QVC
Studio Park
West Chester, PA 19380
(800) 345-1515

Gaia Herbs
108 Island Ford Road
Brevard, NC 28712
(800) 831-7780

Genisoy Products Co.
Fairfield, CA 94533
(888) 436-4769

Health from the Sun
POB 840
Sunapee, NH 03782

Himalaya USA
(800) 869-4640

Hyland's Homeopathics
R and S Laboratories
Los Angeles, CA 90061
(800) 624-9659

Madis Botanicals, Inc.
375 Huyler Street
South Hackensack, NJ 07606
(201) 440-5000

Materia Medica, Inc.
112 Hermosa SE
Albuquerque, NM 87108
(505) 232-3161

Medicine from Nature
10 Mountain Springs Parkway
Springville, VT 84663

Natra-Bio (Homeopathics)
Ferndale, WA 98248
(360) 384-5656

Nature's Way
10 Mountain Springs Parkway
Springfield, UT 84664
(801) 489-1500

Nutra Soy
Narula Research
107 Boulder Bluff Trail
Chapel Hill, NC 27516
(919) 967-7621

Prevail
2204-8 NW Birdsale
Gresham, OR 97030
(800) 248-0885

Transitions for Health
621 SW Alder
Portland, OR 97205
(800) 888-6814

Vitanica
POB 1285
Sherwood, OR 97140
(800) 572-4712

Wise Woman
POB 279
Cresswell, OR 97426
(800) 532-5219

For Licensed Health-Care Practitioners Only

Bezwecken
15495 SW Millikan Way
Beaverton, OR 97006
(800) 743-2256

Ethical Nutrients
(800) 638-2848

Maharishi Ayur-Ved
(800) 826-8424

Metagenics
1010 Tyinn Street #26
Eugene, OR 97402
(800) 338-3948

NF Formulas
9775 SW Commerce Circle
Suite C-5
Wilsonville, OR 97070

Phytopharmica
825 Challenger Drive
Green Bay, WI 54311
(800) 553-2370

Priority One
715 West Orchard
Bellingham, WA 98225
(800) 443-2039

Pure Encapulations
490 Boston Post Road
Sudburg, MA 01776
(800) 753-2277

Scientific Botanicals
POB 31131
Seattle, WA 98103
(206) 527-5521

Thorne Research
25820 Highway 2W
POB 25
Dover, ID 83825
(800) 228-1966

Tyler Encapulations
2204 North Birdsdale
Gresham, OR 97030
(503) 661-5401

Laboratories That Perform the Salivary Hormone Assay

Aeron LifeCycles Clinical Laboratory
1933 Davis Street, Suite 310
San Leandro, CA 94577
(877) 442-3766

Diagnos-techs, Inc.
POB 58948
Scottsdale, AZ 98138-1948
(800) 878-8787

Great Smokies Laboratory
63 Zillicoa Street
Asheville, NC 28801
(800) 522-4762

Sabre Sciences
910 Hampshire Road, Suite P
Westlake Village, CA 91361
(888) 490-7300

Referral Sources for Physicians (Alternative, Complementary, and Integrative Medicine)

American Academy of Anti-Aging Medicine
(312) 345-7936

American Association of Naturopathic Physicians
(206) 323-7610

American College for Advancement of Medicine
(800) 532-3688

American Holistic Medical Association
(703) 556-9728

American Preventive Medical Association
(800) 230-2762

Index